Going Places in Northern Europe

Armchair Adventures and Activities

Gloria Hoffner, BA, AC-BC, ADC, CDP

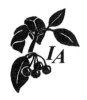

Idyll Arbor, Inc.

39129 264th Ave SE, Enumclaw, WA 98022 (360) 825-7797

Idyll Arbor Editor: Sandra Swenby
Cover design: Curt Pliler

ISBN: 9781882883981

Printed in the United States of America

DEDICATION

To my parents Gloria and George Hoffner who encouraged learning and paid my tuition, to the dedicated Sisters and teachers at St. Madeline School and Cardinal O'Hara High School for giving me a love of writing, world history, geography, and culture, and to my wonderful husband Jim, my partner in traveling the world.

CONTENTS

Acknowledgements vii

Introduction 1

How to Use This Book 3

Austria .... *Oct 7* 13

Belgium 33

Denmark 53

England 73

Finland 93

France ...... *Sept 26* 113

Germany .... *Oct 24 Beer Tasting* 135

Iceland 157

Ireland 175

Luxembourg 197

Netherlands 215

Northern Ireland 235

Norway 255

Scotland 275

Sweden 297

Switzerland 317

Wales 337

ACKNOWLEDGEMENTS

My deep thanks to my loving family — sisters Helen and Nancy, brother-in-law Tony, sons Richard and Stephen, nephew Ryan and niece Nicole — all true blessings in my life.

To Sterling Healthcare and Rehabilitation Center (Media, Pennsylvania) activity director Nancy Newman, general manager Frank Marchese, and the activity department staff.

To my very supportive friends and fellow "newspaper gal reporters" Mary Anne Janco, Barbara Ormsby, Linda Reilly, and Maggie Clark Miller.

Northern Europe

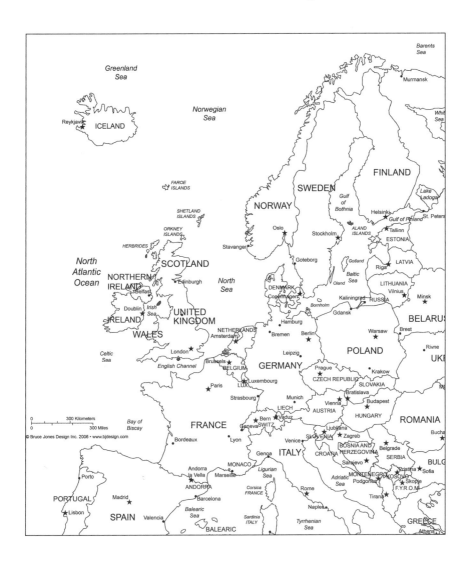

INTRODUCTION

Those faraway places with the strange sounding
names are calling, calling me...
— Far Away Places, lyrics by Joan Whitney and
Alex Kramer.

So say our hearts and minds when we open ourselves to learning about new places on the planet. These places are filled with people of those faraway lands and their history, traditions, culture, and recipes.

Activity directors live in a multicultural world and work in multiple facilities ranging from independent retirement communities to long-term care and from senior community centers to dementia residences and adult day programs. In each there may be residents, clients, and staff from many different places on the globe.

There are many benefits to including programs on foreign lands in your activity offerings.

A travel program allows the activity staff to connect with the memories of residents who lived in another country, have friends or relatives overseas, or who enjoyed traveling in their youth. It improves the connection between staff, which may have been born in a foreign land, and the senior Americans they serve every day.

In March 2000 the estimated number of foreign-born people age 65 and older in the US was 3.1 million. Latin American and Asian immigrants currently represent 53 percent of all immigrants. These two groups now comprise 31 and 22 percent of the older, foreign-born, US population, respectively. By 2050 the Census Bureau estimates that the US population will be 420 million due to a projected 30 percent immigration increase, yielding a racial and ethnic distribution of 50 percent white non-Hispanic, 14 percent Black, 24 percent Hispanic, eight percent Asian, and four percent other.

Discovering other countries improves brain function through learning new information. Keith L. Black, M.D., chair of neurosurgery at Cedars-Sinai Medical Center in Los Angeles, said, "When you challenge your brain you increase the number of brain cells and the connections between those cells. It's not enough to do things you routinely do, like the daily crossword. You have to learn new things."

Cynthia Green, author of the book *Thirty Days to Total Brain Health*, said, "Engaging the mind can help older brains maintain healthy functioning." She added that watching videos of foreign lands provides visual and sensory stimulation by showing residents the natural and manmade beauty of the planet. It is enhanced when accompanied by letting them see, feel, and taste food from other lands.

Benefits of Travel Programs

Travel programs work with residents of all ages and all cognitive and physical abilities in long-term care as well as short-term rehabilitation, and include International Classification of Health Interventions (ICHI) benefits.

Travel programs can involve family members in an ongoing residential activity program.

Travel programs are inexpensive. Activity departments can borrow free videos from the local library or show videos from YouTube and other online services, recruit free speakers, and incorporate recipes into the existing monthly menu.

Travel programs can be used as daily, weekly, monthly, or even annual activities.

Travel programs can be intergenerational, inviting school-age ethnic dance and music groups to visit and entertain residents.

Travel programs serve both current and future long-term residents — the baby boomers are the best traveled and most diverse Americans in US history.

HOW TO USE THIS BOOK

Each chapter in this book discusses a country in Northern Europe — Austria, Belgium, Denmark, England, Finland, France, Germany, Iceland, Ireland, Luxembourg, Netherlands, Northern Ireland, Norway, Scotland, Sweden, Switzerland, and Wales. Each chapter covers the country's geography, language, national holidays, history, travel options, American roots, music and dance, food, and customs. Trivia questions for residents to answer are scattered throughout.

DVD and online video suggestions for showing images and culture are included for each country. Activity directors can find additional online videos concerning cultural and current events via websites such as Netflix, Hulu, Amazon, Discovery Channel, Travel Channel, National Geographic, History Channel, YouTube, and CNN.

This book is designed to be used for a travel activity lasting one hour, one day, or one week, and spread over daily, weekly, monthly, or annual sessions. It can provide new ways to celebrate special events, such as holidays including St. Patrick's Day and Bastille Day.

Each chapter's Game section includes a fun and easy traditional game and a list of the cognitive and physical benefits of participation as outlined by the International Classification of Functioning, Disability, and Health (ICF) and by the guidelines of the International Classification of Health Interventions (ICHI).

Suggestions for one-hour travel-themed fun

Trivia over the morning coffee hour. Once a week or once a month list a country as the discussion topic on your activity calendar. Begin by asking, "Who has traveled to this country?" and "Who has relatives or ancestors from this country?" Then use this book's trivia questions for the country of choice.

After-lunch art activity. Using the website suggestions in each chapter of this book, print a country's flag or map and place it in the center of each dining table — without naming where it is from. Tell residents to bring the flag/map with them to the after-lunch activity. Begin with a guessing game about which country is represented by the flag/map. Once guessed, give everyone a flag/map to color or draw on as inspiration for an art program.

Mid-morning or mid-afternoon music and exercise. Shake up the exercise program by chair dancing to the music of a new country once a month. Using the music videos suggested in this book, add simple arm and leg movements to the rhythm of the music.

Afternoon delights. In the afternoon, bake a dessert or prepare another recipe in this book to be enjoyed with dinner. Preparing the food is an activity that involves fine motor skills, counting, and working as a group. Post the name of the country and the special treat on the dining room menu so residents can see it when they arrive for dinner.

After-dinner learning activity. Use the geography, history, and language information in this book to hold a discussion about the country. Ask residents, "How is the geography of this country the same or different from our country, from where you grew up, or from where your children live?" Discuss how the history of the people reminds them of the struggles and achievements of other cultures.

Last activity of the day: a card game. Use the games in this book to play a card game such as Snap from Ireland or Spoons from England.

A Full Day of Travel or Holiday Activities

Start the day over coffee and use the trivia in this book to allow residents to learn where they will be spending an imaginary travel day. Let's use Ireland as an example. You could ask, "Why is the shamrock the symbol of Ireland?" Residents will learn the size, the language, and the favorite sports of the land via trivia questions.

After coffee. Play a game found in this book, for example, the Irish card game Snap.

At lunch. Place a question about Ireland on every table or place one question on the dining room menu. Invite residents to come to the afternoon cooking event with their best answers. The person with the best answer wins a prize.

After lunch. Use the video suggestions in this book to show and discuss famous landmarks in Ireland. Ask residents who has visited Ireland and/or who has relatives from Ireland.

In the afternoon. Use the recipe in this book to bake Irish scones to be served after dinner.

At dinner. Place the name of a famous person from Ireland, such as St. Patrick, on every dining table. Tell residents to come to the after-dinner activity to learn about this person and how they became famous.

After dinner. Use the trivia questions in this book for a "Who's Who" challenge to teach residents about the famous people of Ireland and their contributions to the world.

End the evening with art and music. Use online suggestions in this book to play Irish music while residents are free to draw an image of anything they learned that day about Ireland.

A Week of Travel Activities

Sunday. Make travel plans to kick off the week. At the morning coffee session tell residents your imaginary trip destination. Use this book to show how long it will take to travel to your destination, where you will stay, and what famous landmarks you will visit. Engage residents with photos downloaded from suggested websites in this book and have those who have visited the country tell their travel stories. In the afternoon, they can make their own travel passports/journals with simple construction paper to record their imaginary trip adventures.

Monday. An afternoon of music. Using suggested websites from this book, play music from the country and show native dancers. Have residents chair-dance to the music! Ask residents how the music makes them feel, how the instruments used are the same or different from their own country's, etc.

Tuesday. Taste of travel. Use the recipe in this book to make a food from the country you are visiting. As the food cooks, use the food trivia in this book to learn about different menu and cooking styles. Serve the food at the end of the day while residents watch images and videos of places in the country from the suggested websites of places in the country.

Wednesday. History on parade. Using the trivia in this book, give every resident the name of a famous person and the reason they are famous. Seat residents in a circle and have them take turns saying who they are and asking other residents to guess what they did to make them famous. For residents unable to read, the activity leader can say, "Martha's (the name of the resident) famous person is Albert Einstein. What did he do?" Residents win if no one guesses. Then the activity leader can give the answer.

Thursday. Draw the world. Use the suggested websites to print out a flag or map of the country and have residents complete the image or draw something of their own choosing to represent the country. Have everyone tell what they drew and why. It's also a great time for the activity leader to tell residents about the history, geography, and language of the country. You can save the maps, drawings, and pictures of the country in scrapbooks for each resident. That will help the residents remember the countries and give them a way to show to their visitors the countries they have discovered through armchair travel.

Friday. Games people play. Host a game tournament using a game from the country. Seat residents at tables and follow the game instructions in this book.

Saturday. Differences delight. End the week with a lively discussion of country customs. How are weddings celebrated in the US as compared to the country visited? What customs from other countries are also traditions in America? Have residents remember their own weddings, their family's weddings, and fun stories. What have they learned about the country this week that surprised them, that gave them something to ponder, and that they never knew before this week?

A Weekly or Monthly Travel Day

Pick a day each week or month to be, for example, Travel Thursday or Travel August. List this on the activity calendar with a "?" and the time for the event.

Have music from the country playing when residents arrive and ask them to guess where they will be visiting today.

Open the activity with fun trivia from this book about the country

Make a recipe found in the book.

After lunch, draw or color a flag or map from the country.

At dinner, put a famous-person trivia question on every table. After dinner, invite residents to play a game. Then answer the trivia question and play a traditional game from the country.

Even More Ideas

International holidays. Add these dates to your monthly activity calendar, for example, national holidays such as St. David's Day in Wales and International Workers' Day in Germany.

Homeland. Select the homeland of a resident and use it as the theme for a day of activities. On the calendar or on a white board at the entrance to the activity room, list "Today we are visiting Rosa's homeland — Iceland."

Customs. Select one fun topic, such as weddings or the games people play, and use it to discover customs from many countries. For example: discuss wedding traditions in five European countries over coffee and cake or host an afternoon tournament of card games from the United Kingdom.

Music and memory game. Play music from different countries such as an Irish Jig and the Hora of Romanian Jews and ask residents to guess where the music originated.

Who am I? Use the *American Roots* sections of this book to provide daily trivia from around the world.

Birthdays. Use the recipes to celebrate residents' birthdays by making a food from their native land or hosting an international food festival for residents and families.

Clubs. Use the reference section of the book to start an international book and coffee club.

Current events. Use the location, language, and history of each country to enhance discussions of ongoing worldwide current events. This book includes the distance from major US cities to each country. You can further personalize this by going online to TravelMath.com and typing in the name of your nearest airport for the distance to your hometown.

Images and videos. Use the internet as a source of photos and videos. For example, search youtube.com for what you are seeking, for example, "Irish folk music" or "German traditional dances" and review the results for use in your programming.

Plan a trip. Working with residents who are independent, in short-stay rehabilitation, or anyone experienced in travel, you can use the suggested hotels and landmarks in this book to plan a group trip or allow them to choose their own trip by using websites such as Tripadvisor.com, Expedia.com, and Hotels.com. Residents can browse through options online to plan an imaginary trip of luxury-only hotels or all-elder hostels. They can select a vacation filled with outdoor adventures such as the best places to fish or an all-spa tour!

This is an opportunity for residents to seek out and plan their perfect get-away. Do they want a vacation filled with visits to famous monuments or do they want to concentrate on natural landscapes? Do residents enjoy sampling local foods or do they like finding shops with unique souvenirs?

Website suggestions. These website suggestions will let residents map out an armchair trip that fits their personality and interests.

www.gearjunkie.com This website can show you the best places to hike throughout the world, from the US to Nepal.

www.lhw.com This website lists the leading hotels of the world and can show you the best places to stay anywhere in the world.

www.lonelyplanet.com This website can show you places of natural beauty, wildlife, adventure, and food and drink from around the world.

www.nationalgeographicexpeditions.com This website can show you incredible views of locations around the world and offers trips accompanied by a trained guide to give you information on the location.

www.roadscholar.org This website lists 5,000 educational tour packages in 150 countries.

www.theworlds50best.com This website lists the world's 50 best restaurants and can show you where to eat like royalty.

www.travelandleisure.com This website's feature articles can give you insights on the best places to dine around the world. It even has information on where famous people vacation.

www.travelmath.com This website let you see the distance from your location to anywhere in the world, both in miles and in traveling time.

www.tripadvisor.com This website lets you compare the prices of hotel rooms and also lets you read reviews from recent travelers, which give real-life information such as the condition of the hotel swimming pool or the convenience and view from a fourth-floor suite.

www.youramazingplaces.com This website can show you travel, art, architecture, and photography from around the world.

Topics and Activities

This book is divided by country and then by topic, each topic containing trivia and a corresponding activity.

Geography, Language, History, and Travel. Residents will color maps and flags of the country.

American Roots. Residents will answer trivia questions and test their knowledge of famous people from the country and Americans whose ancestral roots go back to the country.

Sports and Games. Residents will play a game from the country and answer trivia questions.

Music and Dance. Residents will listen to music, view suggested dance videos, and answer trivia questions.

Food. Residents will learn fun food facts and cook a recipe from the country.

Customs. Residents will compare wedding and children's customs between countries, learn national holidays, and have fun with trivia questions.

Getting Started

Take an inventory of residents' and staff's home countries.

Find out who would love to speak about, share photos of, or contribute a recipe from their native land.

Select a country.

Choose an activity.

Preview video and music to ensure appropriate material and length.

Test a recipe.

Holidays

Winter Holidays. January, February, and March

January 1. New Year's Day in all countries.
January 6. Epiphany in Sweden, Finland, and Austria.
First Monday in February. Winter Holiday in Scotland.
February 14. St. Valentine's Day in Wales.
March 1. St. David's Day, patron saint of Wales.
March 17. St. Patrick's Day in Ireland and Northern Ireland.
Third Sunday in March. Mothering Sunday in Wales.
Variable date. Shrove Tuesday in Wales.
Variable date. Maundy Thursday in Norway.
Variable date. Good Friday in Sweden, Germany, Northern Ireland, England, Scotland, Wales, France, Germany, Switzerland, Denmark, and Belgium.
Variable date. Easter in all countries.
Variable date. Easter Monday in all countries.

Spring Holidays. April and May

April 23. First Day of Summer in Iceland.
April 27. King's Birthday in the Netherlands.
Variable date (day after Pentecost). Whit Monday in Luxembourg, Netherlands, Iceland, France, Finland, Norway, Switzerland, Austria, and Denmark.
May 1. May Day in France, Finland, and Norway.
May 1. Great Prayer Day in Denmark.
May 1. Labor Day in Austria, Scotland, Iceland, Sweden, and Luxembourg.
May 1. International Worker's Day in Germany.
First Monday in May: May Day in Ireland, Northern Ireland, and England.
May 8. Victory in Europe Day in France.
May 10. Mother's Day in Finland.
Variable date. Ascension Day in Denmark, Austria, Iceland, Sweden, Luxembourg, Finland, Norway, and Belgium.
May 17. Constitution Day in Norway.

May 25. Victoria Day in Scotland.
Last Monday in May. Spring Break in Northern Ireland.

Summer Holidays. June, July, and August

First Monday in June. June Holiday in Ireland.
June 4. Corpus Christi in Austria.
June 5. Constitution Day in Denmark.
June 6. National Day in Sweden.
June 17. Icelandic Republic Day in Iceland.
Third Sunday in June: Father's Day in Wales.
June 19. Midsummer Eve in Sweden.
June 20. Midsummer Eve in Finland.
June 21. Belgium National Day in Belgium.
June 23. National Holiday in Luxembourg.
June 23. Midsummer Eve in Norway.
July 12. Orangeman's Day in Northern Ireland.
First Monday in August. August Holiday in Ireland.
July 14. Bastille Day in France.
August 1. Swiss National Day in Switzerland.
August 8. Peace Festival in Germany.
August 15. Assumption Day in Luxembourg and Austria.
Last Monday in August. Summer Bank Holiday in Northern Ireland, Wales, and England.

Fall Holidays. September, October, and November

Last Monday in September. Autumn Holiday in Scotland and Wales.
October 3. German Unity Day in Germany.
October 26. National Day of Austria in Austria.
October 31. Reformation Day in Germany.
October 31. All Saints Day in Sweden and Finland.
Last Monday in October. October Holiday in Ireland.
November 1. All Saints Day in Austria.
November 8. Father's Day in Sweden.
November 11. Armistice Day in Belgium and France.

End-of-year Holidays. December

December 6. Independence Day in Finland.

December 25. Christmas in all.

December 26. St. Stephen's Day in Luxembourg, France, Germany, Ireland, Finland, and Switzerland.

December 26. Boxing Day in Sweden, Northern Ireland, Scotland, England, Norway, and Wales.

December 26. Second Day of Christmas in Netherlands and Iceland.

December 31. New Year's Eve in all.

AUSTRIA

Basics

Geography

Austria is a landlocked country situated in south-central Europe and, at 32,000 square miles, is slightly smaller than the US state of Maine. It is bordered by Germany, the Czech Republic, Italy, Slovenia, Hungary, Switzerland, Slovakia, and Liechtenstein. Over one-third of the country is forested and the lake fishing industry employs over 16,000 people.

The country's natural resources include iron ore, crude oil, magnetite, salt, and zinc ore. Other commercially mined products include copper, lead, antimony, bauxite, tungsten, and natural gas. Austria has numerous hydroelectric installations, which together produce nearly two-thirds of the country's electrical output.

Language

The official language of Austria is German. Other languages spoken in the country include Czech, Sinte Romani, Slovak, Austro-Bavarian, and Alemannic.

History

The history of Austria began in the Danube valley and the Alpine valleys where researchers believe people were living by 8000 BC. In about 400 BC Celtic peoples from Western Europe settled in the eastern Alps. The Romans arrived in 200 BC and by 15 BC they controlled the area.

Germans arrived about 200 AD and through various dynasties, the last being the Habsburg, remained through the twentieth century.

In June 1914 the assassination of the Austrian archduke Franz Ferdinand and Austria's declaration of war against Serbia began World War I. Emperor Franz Joseph died in 1916 and after the end of the war in 1918 the first Republic of Austria was established, ending the 640-year-old Habsburg dynasty.

In 1932 Engelbert Dollfuss became chancellor and in May 1934 he declared martial law in order to protect Austria from Hitler. In July 1934 Dollfuss was shot and killed by Nazis in an attempted coup.

On March 12, 1938, German troops marched into Austria and the country was incorporated into the German Reich ruled by Adolf Hitler. After the end of World War II in 1945, Austria's 1937 frontiers were restored and Austria was occupied by the victorious Allies until 1955 when its sovereign status was restored. In 1995 Austria became a member of the European Union.

Map and Flag

Printable map for coloring and crafts. Accessed January 14, 2015,
  http://www.enchantedlearning.com/europe/austria/outlinemap
Printable flag for coloring. Accessed March 13, 2015,
  http://www.morecoloringpages.com/austria-flag_2468.html

Travel

Distance

From New York, NY, to Vienna, Austria, is 4,234 miles. Flight time is 8 hours 58 minutes.

From Chicago, IL, to Vienna is 4,698 miles. Flight time is 9 hours 54 minutes.

From Dallas, TX, to Vienna is 5,502 miles. Flight time is 11 hours 30 minutes.

From Anchorage to Vienna is 4,854 miles. Flight time is 10 hours 12 minutes.

Hotels

Boutique Hotel Am Dom. Located in Salzburg, a converted 800-year-old town house with modern decor.

Haus St. Benedikt. Located in Salburg. Although primarily the home of young novices in training to become Benedictine monks, guests are welcome. Rooms are sparse but include WiFi. Breakfast is self-service and eaten with the monks.

Hollmann Beletage. A modern hotel located in Vienna which features apartment-style suites with fireplaces.

Hotel Imperial. Opened in Vienna in 1873, it features massive suites and marble floors.

Hotel Schloss Monchstein. Located in Salzburg, its windows overlook the city and an excellent spa.

Landmarks

Benedictine Convent on Nonnberg. Located in Salzburg, it was used as the convent in *The Sound of Music*.

Hofburg. A castle/palace in Vienna dating back to the thirteenth century, it was the formal palace of the Hapsburgs.

Leopoldskron Palace. Located in Salzburg, it was the setting for the Von Trapp Family house in *The Sound of Music*.

Schönbrunn Palace. The summer home of the Hapsburgs, surrounded by beautiful gardens.

St. Charles's Church. Considered one of the finest examples of Baroque architecture in Vienna.

St. Stephen's Cathedral. Located in Vienna, visitors can climb the south tower for an incredible view of the city.

Vitalberg-Steinol Museum. Located in Pertisau in a beautiful setting in the Alps, it houses natural history exhibits going back hundreds of years.

Travel Trivia

What is the official name of Austria?
The Republic of Austria.

What is the capitol of Austria?
Vienna.

What is the German name for Austria?
Eastern Empire, because Austria was once part of the Holy Roman Empire.

True or false: Austria is a member of NATO.
False: It is the only European Union country that is not a member.

What is the highest mountain in Austria?
Grossglockner is the highest mountain in Austria and the second highest in the Alps.

What present-day countries were part of the sixteenth-century Austrian Empire?
Austria, Belgium, Czechoslovakia, Hungary, the Netherlands, Spain, parts of Italy, and the former Yugoslavia.

What is Schonbrunn Palace?
The summer home of the Habsburgs, which has over 1,440 rooms.

Where is the Pasteze Glacier?
Located in the Austrian Alps, it is one of largest glaciers in Europe.

What are the Krimml Falls?
One of the highest waterfalls in Europe.

Name a natural lake in Austria.
The largest is Lake Neusiedler.

What is the Semmering Railway?
The mountain railway running over the Semmering pass between Gloggnitz and Mürzzuschlag is considered one of the greatest civil engineering works of the nineteenth century.

Where is the oldest zoo in the world?
Tiergarten Schönbrunn in Vienna, founded in 1752.

True or false: There are more dead people in Vienna than living residents.
True. The city's Central Cemetery has over 2.5 million tombs.

Name some famous residents of Central Cemetery.
Beethoven, Brahms, Gluck, Schubert, Schoenberg, and Strauss.

When was the Austrian flag designed?
In 1191, when Duke Leopold V fought in the Battle of Acre during the Third Crusade.

Where is the world's largest emerald?
The 2,860 carat jewel is in the Imperial Treasury of the Hofburg, the Imperial Palace in Vienna.

Where is the oldest restaurant/inn in the world?
In Haslauer, founded in 803 AD.

How much of Austria is in the Alps?
Sixty-two percent.

How many Austrians live in Vienna?
A quarter of the population.

True or false: Austrians work the shortest work week in Europe.
False: They work the longest, 45 hours.

America's Roots

Name a famous American dancer with Austrian roots.
Fred Astaire, who revolutionized the movie musical with his elegant and seemingly effortless dance style. He was a well-known perfectionist and spent endless hours in practice.

Who was Felix Frankfurter?
Born in Austria-Hungary, he became an Associate Justice of the United States Supreme Court. He graduated from Harvard Law School and helped found the American Civil Liberties Union.

Who is Eric Richard Kandel?
Born in Austria and graduated from Harvard, he is a neuropsychiatrist and the recipient of the 2000 Nobel Prize in Physiology or Medicine for his research on the physiological basis of memory storage in neurons.

Who is Wolfgang Johannes Puck?
Born in Austria and moved to America at age 24, he is a celebrity chef, who owns restaurants, catering services, and cookbooks through the Wolfgang Puck Companies.

Who was Victor Frederick Weisskopf?
Born in Austria-Hungary, this physicist moved to America and worked on the Manhattan Project during World War II to develop the atomic bomb. He later campaigned against the proliferation of nuclear weapons.

Who is Elijah Jordan Wood?
An actor and film producer born in Iowa with ancestors from Austria. As a child, he starred in the films *Radio Flyer*, *The Good Son*, *North*, and *Flipper*.

Who was Max Fleischer?
An American animator, inventor, film director, and producer who was born in Austria-Hungary in 1883. He invented the Rotoscope.

Who was Felix Weihs de Weldon?
An Austrian-born American sculptor who created the Marine Corps War Memorial showing five US Marines and one US sailor raising the US flag on the island Iwo Jima during World War II. He moved to the United States in 1937.

Who was Ludwig Heinrich Edler von Mises?
A philosopher, Austrian School economist, sociologist, and classical liberal who is known for his work on praxeology, the study of human choice and action. Born in Austria-Hungary, he moved to the United states in 1940 to escape the Nazis.

Who was Arthur Murray?
Born in Austria-Hungary, he came to the United States at age 2. He was a businessman and American dance instructor whose students included Eleanor Roosevelt, the Duke of Windsor, and John D. Rockefeller Jr.

Who was Greta Kempton?
Born in Austria, she came to the United States in the 1920s. She was the White House artist during the Truman administration.

Who was David Karfunkle?
Born in Austria, he became an American artist. Known for his mural, *Exploitation of Labor and Hoarding of Wealth*, painted in 1936 at the Harlem Courthouse in New York City.

Who was Godfrey Edward Arnold?
Born in Austria-Hungary and came to the United States in 1949. He was a professor of medicine and researcher of speech and speech disorders.

Who was Ken Uston?
Born in New York City to a family with Austrian roots. A blackjack player, strategist, and author, he is credited with popularizing the concept of team play at blackjack.

Who was Fred Zinnemann?
Born in Austria-Hungary, he moved to the United States in the 1940s where, as a film director, he won four Academy Awards.

Sports and Games

Sports

The most popular sports in Austria are soccer, alpine skiing, and ice hockey. Since a large portion of the country is located in the Alps, snowboarding, ski jumping, bobsledding, luge, and skeleton (a form of sledding) are also popular.

The country has 12 professional ice hockey teams. Austria has been a world leader in alpine skiing in the Winter Olympics, the FIS Alpine World Ski Championships, and the FIS Ski Jumping World Cup.

Away from the snow, Austrians enjoy basketball, rugby, and motorsports. The Austrian Grand Prix is a Formula One race held in 1963, 1964, from 1970 to 1987, from 1997 to 2003, and since 2014. Several Austrian drivers have competed successfully in Formula One.

Sports Trivia

Who is Niki Lauda?
A three-time Austrian Formula One champion in 1975, 1977, and 1984 and seventh-ranked driver, with 25 wins.

Who was Jochen Rindt?
This Formula One driver won in 1965 and was killed in a practice race in 1970.

Who was Adelbert "Del" St. John?
A Canadian-Austrian professional ice hockey player who competed as a member of the Austria men's national ice hockey team at the 1964 and 1968 Winter Olympic Games.

Who was Toni Sailer?
At the 1956 Olympic Games he was the first to win gold in all of the available events in alpine skiing. At age 20 he was the youngest male gold medalist until 2014.

How many winter Olympic medals has Austria won?
Austrian competitors have won a total of 218 medals, including 59 golds.

What year did Austria not compete in the Winter Olympics?
1936.

What unique winter sports record does Austria hold?
At least one Austrian has won an Olympic winter medal every year, except in 1936.

What famous couple was honored at the Youth Olympic Games Ice Dance in 2012?
Simon Eisenbauer and Christine Smith dressed as Emperor Franz Joseph I and his wife Sissi. They placed ninth in the competition.

Name an Austrian bobsledder who competed in the 1960s.
Erwin Thaler won two silver medals in the four-man event at the 1964 and 1968 Winter Olympics and two medals at the FIBT World Championships, gold in the two-man event in 1967 and a bronze in the four-man event in 1963.

Who is Margarita Marbler?
A retired Austrian freestyle moguls skier who competed in the Winter Olympic Games at Salt Lake City, Turin, and Vancouver. She has competed in both the Moguls and Dual Moguls events as well as in the Acrobatics and Aerials events.

Game

Snap ball. A popular outdoor game in Austria, here modified for residents in wheelchairs to play indoors: Divide the residents into two teams and line up in rows across from each other. The activity person tosses a soft indoor ball to one team member. That team member throws to a member of the opposite team. If the opposite player catches the ball, they hand the ball to the person next to them and that person tosses to the other team.

Number of players. As few as four players, two per team, or as many as 20 players, 10 per team. The teams must always have an equal number of players.

Materials. One large soft indoor ball.

Winner. If any person fails to catch the ball, they are out and are removed from the game. The next member of their team throws to the opposing team and this continues until there is one remaining player, who is the winner.

ICHI benefits. Mental function of language, voice and articulation, control of voluntary movements, and mobility of joints.

Music and Dance

Music

Austria has been a mecca for classical music since the 16th Century when the kings welcomed musicians to perform for the royal court.

Joseph Haydn was born in 1732 in Rohrau, Austria, a village near the Hungarian border. He wrote over 300 pieces including the opera *L'anima del filosofo* and the 12 London Symphonies which include the beloved *Drumroll Symphony*. According to music scholars, Haydn incorporated the styles of Hungarian and Croat folk songs into his music.

Johann Strauss the Elder, born in Vienna in 1804, has been called one of the most famous composers of Viennese waltzes. He began his career as a viola player in the dance orchestra owned by Michael Pamer. He wrote eighteen marches, of which the *Radetzky March* became the most popular, and more than 150 waltzes.

Johann Strauss, often referred to as Johann Strauss II, born in Vienna in 1825, wrote more than 500 musical compositions, including 150 waltzes, of which *The Blue Danube* earned him the name "The Waltz King."

Ludwig van Beethoven, born in Germany in 1770, moved to Vienna in 1792 to study with Haydn and remained in Austria until his death. In about 1800 his hearing began to deteriorate, and by the last decade of his life he was almost totally deaf. During this time he wrote *The Ninth Symphony*.

Wolfgang Amadeus Mozart, born in 1756 in Salzburg, Austria, began playing multiple instruments in public at age six. He composed hundreds of musical pieces, including sonatas, symphonies, masses, concertos, and operas. Two of his famous works are the operas *The Marriage of Figaro* and *Don Giovanni.*

Music Videos

Austrian Folk Music. Accessed January 15, 2015,
  https://www.youtube.com/watch?v=4_lyS531Q2I
Austrian Viennese traditional music: Philharmonia Schrammeln: Wiener-Spezialitäten-Marsch. Accessed January 15, 2015,
  https://www.youtube.com/watch?v=8sXG4kx-MFI&list=PL1DCA2504E7B4191A
Glanegg Jugend Festival. Accessed January 15, 2015,
  https://www.youtube.com/watch?v=2aQ36Iou0eA
Strauss Waltzes Medley. Accessed January 15, 2015,
  https://www.youtube.com/watch?v=3HM0vsmfnFc
Vienna Waltzes Medley. Accessed January 15, 2015,
  https://www.youtube.com/watch?v=0-LOkF-oK8o

Dance

Austria is the home of folk dances and is famous for the waltz. The *Landler* is an eighteenth-century couples' dance performed to music in 3/4 time which features hopping, stamping, and sometimes yodeling.

Schihplattler is the folk dance in which the boys slap their thighs and shoes. Traditionally workers were busy farming in the warm months, so dancing became an indoor winter activity.

Austrian folk dancing has its own costume. The women wear a gathered skirt with petticoats called a *dirndl*. The skirt is full to allow easy movement while dancing. The blouse is traditionally white with short, puffed sleeves. Women dancers also wear a hat, knitted stockings, and black shoes.

Male dancers wear *lederhosen*, leather shorts, and a white, open-necked shirt with rolled-up sleeves and a tie, white stockings, and black shoes.

The waltz was developed from German dances in the 1770s and was originally considered too indecent to be danced by young girls. Only married women were allowed to waltz in the years before the French Revolution. The waltz in the modern sense is danced in pairs and is considered to be a relatively fast ballroom dance.

During the Vienna Congress in 1814, the Vienna waltz started to become socially respectable. Several reputable composers, including Josef Lanner and his rivals Johann Strauss the Elder and Johann Strauss the Younger, created endless variations.

There are three common types of waltz: the French, the English, and the Vienna waltz, which is the fastest. There are two types of Vienna waltz: the International style and the American style.

Traditionally, couples dance a waltz at New Year's to celebrate the new year, and the bride and groom waltz on their wedding day to celebrate their new life as a couple.

Dance Videos

Austrian traditional folk dance: Haidauer & Osterwitzer Schuhplattler: Accessed December 29, 2015, https://www.youtube.com/watch?v=b85BaYS0v50

Austrian waltz on ice: Accessed January 15, 2015, https://www.youtube.com/watch?v=N0hW8OnvSVY

Folk dance: Accessed January 15, 2015, https://www.youtube.com/watch?v=Ju9E9yrC8GU

Lesson Vienna Waltz: Accessed December 29, 2015, https://www.youtube.com/watch?v=ZNKmSthl1QE

Viennese waltz on ice: Accessed January 15, 2015, https://www.youtube.com/watch?v=BjLJEuL1g80

Music and Dance Trivia

What is yodeling?
Yodeling is a form of singing which involves repeated changes of pitch during a single note and is traditionally sung in the Alps.

What is a favorite dance band instrument invented in Austria?
The accordion, invented in 1829.

What is Viennese *schrammelmusik*?
Music that combines rural folk songs and urban dance music.

What kind of guitar is used to play *schrammelmusik*?
A double-necked guitar, one neck with 12 strings and the other with six strings. The instrument dates back to the nineteenth century.

What woodwind instrument is part of a folk dance band?
The clarinet.

What instrument was traditionally found in all rural Austrian homes?
The accordion.

True or false: The chicken dance is from Austria.
False.

What happens before the start of a dance in Austria?
The host gives a speech.

How does a night of dancing in Austria end?
With a good-night dance.

Food

Austrian food traditions combine tastes from Italy, Germany, and Hungary because of the influence of many political changes. The most common meats are beef, chicken, pork, and veal.

Austrians prefer a continental-style breakfast of rolls, cold cuts, jam, cheese, juices, and tea or coffee. While the main meal of the day was traditionally at midday, modern society has moved the main meal to the end of the day. A typical lunch is bread with ham and cheese.

The people of Austria love desserts, especially *sachertorte*, a chocolate cake topped with whipped cream and filled with apricot jam. This is a dessert served in Vienna's many and popular coffee houses.

A favorite main meal is *weiner schnitzel*, which is made from veal. It is believed that this dish came from Milan to Vienna during the sixteenth century.

Wine is a popular Austrian drink. In fact, Vienna is the only capitol city in the world where wine grapes are grown within the city limits.

There are also vineyards in the south, east, and Danube sections of the country.

Cheesemaking is an art linked to the history and culture in Bregenzerwald, Austria. This area produces cheese, yogurt, and locally churned butter. The Alpine Dairy Farming Museum in Hittisau features an alpine dairy kitchen set up exactly the way it was used 300 years ago.

Recipe

Sachertorte Cookies. A favorite dessert. Makes 4 dozen cookies.
Ingredients.
1 cup margarine
4 ounces vanilla instant pudding mix
1 egg
2 cups flour
3 tablespoons sugar
⅔ cup apricot preserves
½ cup semi-sweet chocolate chips
3 tablespoons of butter
Preparation. Preheat oven to 325 degrees F. In a large bowl, combine margarine and pudding mix. Beat until light and fluffy. Add egg and blend well. Add flour and mix well. Shape the dough into 1" balls and roll in sugar. Place the balls 2" apart on an ungreased cookie sheet. Make an indentation in the center of each cookie with your thumb.

Bake for 15 to 18 minutes or until firm to the touch. Immediately remove from cookie sheets and cool. When completely cooled, fill each indentation with 1/2 teaspoon preserves. Melt the chocolate and butter in a sauce pan over low heat and mix until smooth. Drizzle this mixture over the cookies.

Food Trivia

What is Austrian hot chocolate made of?
Heavy cream, chocolate, and egg yolk.

What is the most common beer in Austria?
Wheat beer.

What is the most popular soft drink?
Almdudler, flavored with elderflower and herbs.

What do adults sometimes mix into their *Almdudler*?
White wine.

What is *schweinsbraten*?
Roast pork made from the neck, ham, or shoulder of the pig and cooked until the outside is crispy.

What is a *punschkrapfen*?
A small cake similar to a *petit four*. Made of spongy dough filled with rum, chocolate, and jam. Coated with a thick, pink, rum sugar punch glaze, often drizzled with chocolate with a cocktail cherry placed on top.

How do you prepare *weinerschnitzel*?
Tenderize a thin piece of veal by pounding with a mallet, then dip in wheat flour, eggs, and breadcrumbs, and finally fry in butter.

What is *burenwurst*?
A meat-and-bacon sausage served with sweet mustard and a Kaiser roll at Viennese sausage stands.

What are *marillenknodel*?
Potato dumplings filled with apricots, rolled in crumbs, and dusted with powdered sugar.

What is a *paatschinken*?
A thin pancake filled with jam, similar to a *crepe*.

Customs

Weddings

In Austria the groom does not ask her father for the hand of the bride. Instead, he must propose by sending his family and friends to the family of the future bride to ask if the joining is possible. If anyone from either family saw a blind man, a monk, or a pregnant woman before the proposal, the wedding was considered doomed. However, if anyone saw a goat, pigeon, or wolf, tradition suggested this would be a successful marriage.

It was thought to be bad luck to marry a man whose last name starts with the same initial as the bride's last name. And no bride should practice writing her husband's name prior to the marriage.

The most important part of bringing good luck to the marriage was thought to be the choosing of the wedding day. Thursdays, Fridays, and Saturdays are considered unlucky. A popular rhyme stated, "Monday for wealth, Tuesday for health, and Wednesday the best day of all."

It was thought to be bad luck for a bride to make her own wedding dress and, just as in the United States, bad luck for the groom to see the bride in the dress before the ceremony. Brides were advised not to wear the entire bridal outfit prior to the ceremony, and some even left a stitch to be sewn at the church. The veil's purpose was to protect the bride from evil spirits.

Superstitions even surrounded the flowers at the wedding. Red and white flowers were considered bad luck as they could symbolize blood and bandages. A groom's buttonhole flower must be the same as the flowers in the bride's bouquet.

Bridesmaids' dresses were similar to the bride's to confuse angry spirits.

En route to the wedding, the bride would look in a mirror only once. Looking twice would bring bad luck to her day. A bride who saw a chimney sweep, a spider, a black cat, or a rainbow on the way to the ceremony would have a happy future. Cloudy weather on the wedding day was considered bad luck, but seeing snow meant future fertility for the couple.

Children

Austrian parents celebrate their child's birthday with a party or by going out to dinner. Adults celebrate their birthdays by inviting friends to dinner, paid for by the birthday person.

Holidays

January 1. New Year's Day.
Date varies. Easter.
Date varies. Easter Monday.

Date varies (the day after Pentecost). Whit Monday.
May 1. Labor Day.
Date varies. Ascension Day.
June 4. Corpus Christi Day.
August 15. Assumption Day.
October 26. National Day of Austria.
November 1. All Saints Day.
December 25. Christmas.
December 31. New Year's Eve.

Customs Trivia

How must you step into a house?
With your right foot first. Stepping in with your left foot first is bad luck.

What should you not do at a funeral?
Ride behind a bobtailed horse. If you do, you will have bad luck.

True or false: Sneezing during a full moon is considered bad luck?
True.

What is a cure for the common cold?
Eating sliced raw garlic mixed with yogurt.

True or false: To bring good luck, a man should own a white horse, white cat, white cow, and white umbrella?
These bring bad luck and others are warned not to associate with such a person.

True or false: A girl who sits on a cold sidewalk will become sick.
False:

True or false: Bragging about good fortune will bring you more good luck.
False:

How can you make sure good luck will not leave you?
Knock on nearby wood to drive away the evil spirits hiding in the wood.

What does it mean when you see a relative in a dream?
It means something bad will happen to them.

What does it mean if you see a dead relative in a dream?
It means they need prayers to get into heaven.

More Resources

DVDs

Cities of the World (Austria), DVD. www.travelvideostore.com, 2009.
Globe Trekker: Vienna, DVD. Pilot Productions, 2004.
Passport to Europe: Germany, Switzerland and Austria, DVD.
     www.travelchannel.com, 2007.
Spain, Switzerland, & Austria, DVD. Questar, 2011.
Travel to Austria, DVD. Select Media, 2011.

Books

Bley, E, *Austria in Pictures* (Minneapolis: Lerner, 1991).
Brook-Shephard, G. *The Austrians: A Thousand-Year Odyssey* (New
     York: Carroll & Graf, 2002).
DK Publishing. *DK Eyewitness Travel Guide: Austria* (London: DK
     Publishing, 2014).
Lengyel, E. *The Danube* (New York: Random House, 1939).
Schenk, E. *Mozart and His Times* (New York: Knopf, 1959).

Websites

Austrian Tourism Board: Accessed March 13, 2015,
     http://www.austria.info/us.
Federal Chancellery of Austria: Accessed March 13, 2015,
     https://www.bka.gv.at/site/3327/Default.aspx
Map of Austria: Accessed January 14, 2015,
     http://www.lonelyplanet.com/maps/europe/austria
Maps of the World. Flag of Austria:Accessed March 13, 2015,
     http://www.mapsofworld.com/flags/austria-flag.html
US Department of State. Austria: Accessed March 13, 2015,
     http://www.austria.info/us

Photos

National Geographic photos of Austria: Accessed January 16, 2015,
   http://travel.nationalgeographic.com/travel/countries/austria-photos-traveler
Photobucket Austria: Accessed January 16, 2015,
   http://photobucket.com/images/austria?page=1
Planetware Austria: Accessed January 16, 2015,
   http://www.planetware.com/pictures/austria-a.htm
Rolf Hicker Photos: Accessed January 16, 2015,
   http://www.hickerphoto.com/photos/austria-pictures.htm
Trip Advisor Austria: Accessed January 16, 2015,
   http://www.tripadvisor.com/LocationPhotos-g190410-Austria.html

References

10 Best Austrian Female Singers: Accessed January 15, 2015,
   http://www.mademan.com/mm/10-best-australian-female-singers.html#ixzz3Ow1Yhttn
ATV (Austria): Accessed January 16, 2015, en.wikipedia.org/wiki/ATV_(Austria)
Austria: Accessed January 15, 2015, http://www.dance-kids.org/dancingglobe/austria.html
Austria: Accessed January 14, 2015,
   http://www.nationsencyclopedia.com/economies/Europe/Austria.html#ixzz3Opn6hmoi
Austria Fun Facts: Accessed January 16, 2015,
   http://austriafun.facts.co/funaustriafactsforkids/austriafunfacts.php
Austria's Best Video Collection: Accessed January 16, 2015,
   http://www.austria.info/us/austria-videos
Austria's History: Accessed January 14, 2015, http://www.austria.info/us/about-austria/history-1140682.html
Austrian American: Accessed March 13, 2015,
   https://en.wikipedia.org/wiki/Austrian_American
Austrian Cuisine: Accessed January 16, 2015,
   http://www.aboutaustria.org/recipes/recipes.htm
Austrian Cuisine: Accessed January 16, 2015,
   http://www.worldwidewebawards.net/Food/Austria.html
Austrian Folk Dance: Accessed January 15, 2015,
   http://en.wikipedia.org/wiki/Austrian_folk_dance
Austrian Folk Instruments: Accessed January 15, 2015,
   http://www.ehow.com/list_6820527_austrian-folk-instruments.html
Austrian Games for Children: Accessed January 15, 2015,
   http://www.ehow.com/info_8604484_austrian-games-children.html

Austrian Superstitions: Accessed March 13, 2015,
http://www.latinabroad.com/2012/03/19/austrian-superstitions-part-12-of-the-
worlds-superstitions-series

Austrian Weddings: Accessed January 16, 2015, http://7baustria7.weebly.com/austrian-
weddings.html

Austria's Music History: Accessed January 15, 2015, http://www.austria.info/in/art-
culture/music-history-austria-2200576.html

Best Places to Visit in Austria: Accessed January 16, 2015,
http://www.thereareplaces.com/newguidebook/pdest/aupts.htm

Christmas Traditions around the World: Accessed January 14, 2015,
http://www.santas.net

Coffeehouse Culture in Austria: Accessed January 16, 2015,
http://www.austria.info/us/people-and-traditions/coffeehouse-culture-in-austria-
1145698.html

Courting Vienna: Accessed January 16, 2015,
http://travel.nationalgeographic.com/travel/city-guides/vienna-traveler

Erwin Thaler: Accessed January 15, 2015, http://www.digplanet.com/wiki/Erwin_Thaler

Facts about Austria: Accessed January 16, 2015,
http://lifestyle.iloveindia.com/lounge/facts-about-austria-1592.html

Famous Musicians in Austria's History: Accessed January 15, 2015,
http://german.answers.com/music/famous-musicians-in-austrias-history

Figure Skaters and Ice Dancers from Austria: Accessed January 15, 2015,
http://www.goldenskate.com/directories/skater-directory/figure-skaters-and-ice-
dancers-from-austria

Franz Lizst Biography. Accessed January 15, 2015,
http://www.imdb.com/name/nm0006172/bio

Fred Astaire Biography: Accessed January 15, 2015, www.biography.com/people/fred-
astaire-9190991

Holidays: Accessed January 14, 2015, http://www.timeanddate.com/holidays

Holidays in Austria: Accessed January 16, 2015, https://www.youtube.com/user/austria

Interesting Facts about Austria: Accessed January 14, 2015,
http://www.eupedia.com/austria/trivia.shtml

Johann Strauss Biography: Accessed January 15, 2015,
www.biography.com/people/johann-strauss-9496950

Joseph Haydn: Accessed January 15, 2015,
http://en.wikipedia.org/wiki/Joseph_Haydn#Early_life

Languages of the World. Austria: Accessed January 14, 2015,
http://www.ethnologue.com/country/AT

List of Olympic medalists in alpine skiing: Accessed January 15, 2015,
https://en.wikipedia.org/wiki/List_of_Olympic_medalists_in_alpine_skiing

Ludwig van Beethoven: Accessed January 15, 2015,
http://en.wikipedia.org/wiki/Ludwig_van_Beethoven

Margarita Marbler: Accessed January 15, 2015,
http://www.ranker.com/review/margarita-marbler/18851928

Public National Holidays: Accessed January 14, 2015,
http://www.nationalholidayslist.com

Sport in Austria: Accessed January 14, 2015,
http://en.wikipedia.org/wiki/Sport_in_Austria

Theater Museum Wien: Accessed January 15, 2015,
http://www.tourmycountry.com/austria/theatre-museum-vienna.htm
The History of Austrian Cinema from 1896 to the Present Day: Accessed January 16,
2015,
http://moviemoviesite.com/Countries/Countries%20A/Austria/austria_index.htm
The Hotel Guru: Accessed January 16, 2015, http://www.thehotelguru.com/hotel/haus-st-
benedikt-salzburg
Top 12 Music Festivals in Austria: Accessed January 15, 2015,
http://www.austria.info/us/activities/culture-traditions/music-in-austria/top-12-
music-festivals-in-austria
Top Things to Do in Austrian Alps: Accessed January 16, 2015,
http://www.tripadvisor.com/Attractions-g190434-Activities-Austrian_Alps.html
Travel Guide Austria: Accessed January 16, 2015,
https://www.youtube.com/watch?v=9OLrtATnGWE
Travel Math: Accessed January 16, 2015,
http://www.travelmath.com/from/Anchorage,+AK/to/Vienna,+Austria
Vienna Waltz: The National Dance of Austria: Accessed January 15, 2015,
http://tourmycountry.com/austria/viennawaltz.htm
Wolfgang Mozart Biography: Accessed January 15, 2015,
http://www.biography.com/people/wolfgang-mozart-9417115
Yodeling: Accessed January 15, 2015, http://en.wikipedia.org/wiki/Yodeling

BELGIUM

Basics

Geography

Belgium is located in Western Europe, bordered by the North Sea, France, Germany, Luxembourg, and the Netherlands. Belgium has three main geographical regions: the coastal plain in the northwest, the central plateau, and the Ardennes uplands in the southeast. The coastal plain consists mainly of sand dunes and polders. Polders are areas of land close to or below sea level that have been reclaimed from the sea. These areas are protected by dikes or by fields that have been drained with canals. Belgium's highest point is the Signal de Botrange at 2,277 feet. The country has relatively few natural lakes, and none very large. It is physically about the land size of the US state of Maryland.

Language

There are three official languages: Dutch, French, and German. The country's constitution guarantees freedom of language and minority languages and dialects are often spoken by Belgians. Most Belgians speak more than one language, usually including English.

History

The history of Belgium began with the Belgae, an ancient tribe which lived in the area before the Romans arrived and established the province of Belgica, which was larger than modern Belgium. The Franks first appeared in 3 AD, beginning a series of rulers and dynasties that ended in about 1384 AD when all of present Belgium was ruled by the Dukes of Burgundy.

The country was occupied variously by the Netherlands, Austria, and Spain from 1477 to 1794, then by France during the French Revolutionary Wars and transferred from Austria to France by the Treaty of Campo Formio in 1797. After the defeat of Napoleon at Waterloo in 1815, Belgium was given to the newly formed kingdom of the Netherlands.

The Belgian people rebelled against King William I of the Netherlands in 1830 and Belgian independence was declared. European powers at the London Conference of 1830–31 approved the independence of the nation. In 1831 Prince Leopold of Saxe-Coburg-Gotha was chosen king of the Belgians and became Leopold I.

Under the rule of Leopold II, 1865-1900, Belgium established colonies in the African Congo. During World War I Germany invaded Belgium. After the war, the Treaty of Versailles gave Belgium a mandate over the northwestern corner of former German East Africa.

During World War II, Germany attacked and occupied Belgium in May 1940. In 1960 the Belgian Congo was given its independence.

Map and Flag

Belgium Flag Coloring Page. Accessed April 5, 2015,
   http://www.morecoloringpages.com/belgium-flag_2470.html.
Map of Belgium to Color. Accessed April 5, 2015,
   http://www.hellokids.com/c_1581/coloring-pages/countries-coloring-pages/maps-coloring-pages/belgium-map.

Travel

Distance

Distance from New York, NY, to Brussels is 3,669 miles. Flight time is 7 hours 50 minutes.

Distance from Chicago, IL, to Brussels is 4,150 miles. Flight time is 8 hours 48 minutes.

Distance from Dallas, TX, to Brussels is 4,952 miles. Flight time is 10 hours 24 minutes.

Distance from Seattle, WA, to Brussels is 4,951 miles. Flight time is 10 hours 24 minutes.

Hotels

Die Swaene. Located in Bruges, it features original ceiling paintings and eighteenth-century paneling in the lounge. There is an indoor swimming pool and a sauna.

Hotel Metropole Brussels. Located in Brussels, it is the city's only nineteenth-century hotel still in operation. Furnished in French Renaissance style and architecture and is near the *de grote Markt* (Grand Place), recognized as one of the most beautiful town squares in Europe.

Kempinski Hotel Dukes Palace. Located in Bruges. Although renovated, six rooms have fifteenth-century design charm. There is also a pool, sauna, and gym as well as on-site spa treatments.

Le Chatelain Hotel. Located in Brussels. Features an on-site garden and fitness center as well as many offerings in its on-site restaurant.

Sofitel Brussels Europe. Located in Brussels and offers luxury and modern conveniences including the Sofitel's own *MyBed* designed for comfort and a perfect night's sleep, flat-screen TV, espresso machine, high-speed Internet, WiFi, and a laptop-sized room safe.

Landmarks

Abbaye Notre Dame. A Cistercian monastery since 1132. All but one wall was destroyed during the French Revolution but it was rebuilt so the ancient ruins can still be seen, along with an eighteenth-century pharmacy, medicinal herb garden, and a small museum located in part of the labyrinthine vaults. Interested tourists can sleep in the monastery for two to seven days as part of a spiritual retreat. Guests must join in the daily cycle of prayers and bring their own bed linen.

Brussels Chocolate Walking Tour and Workshop. Guests can learn how to make real Belgian pralines as well as orangettes, pralines, and Easter eggs. During the tour, guests visit *Grand Place*, the former market square, *Manneken Pis*, the iconic statue sculpted by Jerome Duquesnoy in 1619, and *Neuhaus*, the oldest chocolate shop.

Canal Tour. The perfect way to see Bruges. Sailing down *Spiegelrei* towards *Jan Van Eyckplein*, tourists can imagine Venetian merchants entering the city centuries ago and meeting under the slender turret of the *Poortersloge* building.

Citadelle de Namur. A castle in Namur that has ramparts, tunnels, and sections of grey outer wall dating back to medieval times. However, much of the structure was built in the nineteenth and twentieth centuries and still offers wonderful views of the town.

Kattenfestival. Held in Ypres on the second Sunday in May, it began in the twelfth century with a city jester throwing live cats from the *Lakenhalle* belfry because people believed that a cat personified evil spirits. The ritual continued until 1817. Starting in 1930, toy cats are hurled from the belfry for fun. There is also a parade of people dressed up as cats and venders who sell cat-shaped desserts.

World War I Cemetery and Battlefield. Remembered in the poem *In Flanders Fields* written by Canadian Lieutenant Colonel John McCrae in homage to a lost friend. Poppies cover the battlefield and have become the defining floral image of remembrance of the dead. The poppies bloom annually from April to July.

Travel Trivia

True or false: The world's first newspaper was printed in Antwerp, Belgium.
True.

True or false: Belgium legalized euthanasia.
True. Approved in 2002.

True or false: Belgium grants the most new citizenships in the world.
False: The country is second after Canada which grants the most in the world.

True or false: Belgium has the most cars per square mile.
False: Belgium is third after the Netherlands and Japan.

Where was the world's first skyscraper built?
Antwerp, Belgium, in 1928.

True or false: The world's first health spa was in Belgium.
True, established in the eighteenth century.

Who was Sir Eugene Goossens?
A Belgian who led construction of the Sydney (Australia) Opera House.

Where is the smallest town in the world?
Durbuy, Belgium, has just 500 residents.

True or false: Oil painting was invented in Belgium.
True. In the fifteenth century.

Who was Ferdinard Verbiest?
A Belgian Jesuit missionary who invented the first steam-powered car in 1672.

When and where did the first railway line in Europe begin?
On May 5, 1835, between Brussels and Mechelen.

Where is the smallest wage gap between men and women?
Belgium.

Where were Neanderthal skulls first discovered?
Engis, Belgium.

True or false: The Belgium highway system can be seen from the moon.
True, due to the nighttime lighting.

True or false: Belgian householders do not approve of pets.
False: Half of all Belgian homes have at least one pet.

True or false: Belgians have the world's highest use of cable television.
True. Ninety-seven percent have cable.

True or false: There are no discount coupons offered by stores in Belgium.
False: Belgians are the top coupon users in the world.

What is the mandatory school attendance age?
Eighteen.

True or false: Voting is mandatory in Belgium.
True and enforced by law.

True or false: The Belgian airport is the most punctual in the world.
True, according to a 2006 world report.

America's Roots

Who was Hendrick Baekeland?
A Belgian who became a naturalized American and the chemist who invented Velox photographic paper in 1907.

Who was Louis Hennepin?
A Flemish Catholic priest who discovered Niagara Falls and was the first to place Chicago on a map.

Who was Father Damien?
A Flemish missionary who served the lepers in Hawaii.

Who was Charles Stephens?
An American ophthalmologist of Flemish descent who is called the "Father of Modern Retinal Surgery."

Who was George A. Van Biesbroeck?
A Belgian astronomer who came to the US in 1915. He won the Valz Prize for his work studying asteroids and comets.

Who was Henry Ford?
The businessman who created the Ford Motor Company. His mother was from Belgium.

Who was Carl Karcher?
The founder of the American hamburger chain Carl Jr's. He was of Belgian descent.

Who was Jan Yoors?
A Flemish-American artist, painter, and tapestry creator.

Who was George Washington Goethals?
Appointed by US President Theodore Roosevelt to build the Panama Canal, he completed it under budget in 1914. His parents were from Belgium.

Who was Liz Claiborne?
A fashion designer born in Belgium of two American parents.

Who was Charles Joseph Van Depoele?
An electrical engineer and electric railway pioneer born in Belgium who moved to the US in 1869.

Who was Archbishop Charles John Seghers?
Born in Belgium, he came to the United States in 1873 and became the Catholic Bishop of Vancouver (Canada) and Alaska

Who was Maurice Anthony Biot?
A Belgian physicist and the founder of the theory of proelasticity. He moved to the US in 1932.

Who is Karel Bossart?
Born in Belgium, he moved to the US in the 1940s and was a rocket scientist who designed the Atlas ICBM.

Who was Julius Arthur Nieuwland?
A Belgian priest and professor at the University of Notre Dame who helped develop synthetic rubber. He came to the US with his parents in 1880.

Sports and Games

Sports

The most popular sport in Belgium is football, which Americans call soccer. It attracts hundreds of amateurs to local indoor and outdoor clubs and over 25,000 spectators to each professional game.

About 21 percent of Belgians participate in cycling sporting events. The most popular of these is the Tour of Flanders. Famous Belgian cyclists include Eddy Merckx who won the Tour de France five times and Tom Boonen who won the Tour de France green jersey in 2007.

Tennis, not football, attracts the most viewers, 67 percent of Belgium TV viewers compared to football at 51 percent. Two of the country's most famous players are Justine Henin-Hardenne and Kim Clijsters.

Belgians love to run. Over 23 percent of the population participate in track and field events. There are two major marathons in the country: the Antwerp Marathon and the Brussels Marathon. There is also the annual 100 km Nacht van Vlaanderan race.

Other popular sports include basketball, field hockey, swimming, sailing, horseback riding, and golf.

Sports Trivia

Who was Edgard Colle?
A Belgian chess master who pioneered the Colle System.

Who was George Koltanowski?
A chess player and promoter.

Who was Earl Louis "Curly" Lambeau?
The founder, player, and first coach of the US football team Green Bay Packers. He was of Belgian descent.

Who is Roger DeCoster?
A Belgian motorcross racer who has won thirty-six 500cc Grand Prixs.

Who was Art Houtteman?
The youngest baseball player in the American league, from 1945 to 1946. His great grandfather was from Belgium.

Who is Ryan Spilborghs?
A former professional baseball player who is a baseball broadcaster. His father is Belgian.

Who is Kiki Vandeweghe?
A former professional basketball player and the vice president of basketball operations for the National Basketball Association.

Who is Christian Vande Velde?
A professional road cyclist.

Who is John Vanbiesbrouck?
An ice hockey professional goaltender who was inducted into the US Hockey Hall of Fame in 2007. His father is from Belgium.

Where is the oldest golf course on the European continent?
The Royal Golf Course in Tervuren, Belgium, founded in 1906.

Game

Belgian Darts. The game of darts in Belgium began as *vogelpik*, an older game in which players used stuffed birds with needles attached to throw against a board on a wall to gain points. Today the birds have been replaced with feathered darts tossed at a circular target.

Number of players. Two single players or two teams of two players each.

Materials. (modified for residents) four Velcro darts per player and a Velcro dart board.

To play. Each player is given four darts and throws them one after another. The next player does the same. The darts are removed from the board, the score tallied, and the game continues for five rounds.

Winner. The player with the highest score from all five rounds wins.

ICHI benefits. Mental functions of language, articulation and control of voluntary movements, balance, muscle force, and mobility of joints.

Music and Dance

Music

Belgian folk music represents the cultural mix in the country, blending influences from Dutch-speaking Flemish and French-speaking Walloon inhabitants with German minorities and immigrant communities.

Belgian folk music survived the twentieth century due to the efforts of ethnomusicologists. During the 1960s and early 1970s, musicians such as Wannes Van de Velde, Herman Dewit, Walter de Buck, and Hubert Boone led a folk revival. A few of these musicians, especially Van de Velde, modernized Belgian folk music by writing urban songs using influences from Spain and Greece. Wannes, for example, sang in the dialect of his native Antwerp and collaborated with Amparo Cortés, a Spanish flamenco singer.

During the 1970s bands, such as *Rum* and Hubert Boone's influential *Brabants Volksorkest*, modernized traditional folk music. This type of music became less popular in the 1980s, with only a few folk-rock bands, such as *Kadril*, achieving much success. However, Herman Dewit founded an annual music course in Gooik which kept folk music alive. In the mid-1990s, groups such as *Ambrozijn*, *Fluxus*, *Marc Hauman & De Moeite*, and *Laïs* gained fame from these annual folk music events.

Beginning in the 1980s, African musicians became an important part of Belgian music, especially musicians from the former Belgian colony of Congo including Congolese-Belgian Princesse Mansia M'Bila, Rwandan-Belgian Cécile Kayirebwa, and Dieudonné Kabongo. This African influence raised interest in the Argentine tango, Moroccan *oud*, and other music from around the world. The 1990s also saw the emergence of *Zap Mama*, a group of Congolese-Belgian women who played a fusion of Pygmy and other African music with European influences.

Other musical styles, from classical to jazz and popular to hip-hop, can be heard throughout Belgium. Famous classical composers such as Cesar Franck, Henri Vieuxtemps, Guillaume Lekeu, and Wim Mertens were born in Belgium. Well-known singers include pioneer Bobbejaan Schoepen, Johnny Hallyday, Maurane, and Jacques Brel.

Music Videos

20 Hits 20 Singers. Medley Made in Belgium: Accessed April 3, 2015,
    https://www.youtube.com/watch?v=6n2Ls8_tN14
Belgium Folk: Accessed April 3, 2015,
    https://www.youtube.com/watch?v=8epOh-CvcRs
Belgium Music and Images: Accessed April 3, 2015,
    https://www.youtube.com/watch?v=xNx0CP7oQug.
Best Belgium Electro House Music: Accessed April 3, 2015,
    https://www.youtube.com/watch?v=Dcfm43eanFg
European Folk Music Belgium: Accessed April 3, 2015,
    https://www.youtube.com/watch?v=BK0UqTQADoE

Dance

Folk dancing returned as a popular form of art and expression in the late twentieth century. A performance called *balfolk* is popular in many European countries including Belgium. In Flanders, *boombal* is the biggest organization for the popularization of *balfolk*. In fact, this influence is so great that the term *boombal* is used more often than the term *balfolk*.

Balfolk differs from dances by traditional folkdance groups in several ways. Traditional folk dances are extensively choreographed and are often danced wearing traditional clothing with the emphasis on the presentation of tradition. The dance music used may be played live or pre-recorded. The audience sits and watches the dancers perform the dances.

Balfolk dances are generally based on simple traditional choreography so everyone can join in. Refined movements are not the focus and improvisation is common. There are modern music influences, the music is always played by live bands, and the audience participates in the dance.

For those who want to learn, prior to the start of *balfolk* events, workshops for beginning or intermediate dancers are held. In *balfolk* dance partners change during the event. Also, the ages of the dancers ranges from very young to seniors.

Dance Videos

Balfolk tijdens Keltfest: Accessed April 3, 2015,
  https://www.youtube.com/watch?v=yxdhKVZbTFw
Balfolk Utrecht: Wouter Kuyper: Accessed April 3, 2015,
  https://www.youtube.com/watch?v=yxdhKVZbTFw
Belgium Folk Dance: De Loere: Accessed April 3, 2015,
  https://www.youtube.com/watch?v=ZbdU45CueXo
Belgium Folk Dance: Zwierig Dansje: Accessed April 3, 2015,
  https://www.youtube.com/watch?v=y6MxS6SZyvY
Folk Dances from Belgium: Accessed April 3, 2015,
  https://www.youtube.com/watch?v=F75KFD7uiHQ&list=PLD3724
  BE3FBDE6BC9
Summerfest '09. Belgium: Accessed April 3, 2015,
  https://www.youtube.com/watch?v=y6MxS6SZyvY

Music and Dance Trivia

Name a popular Belgium jazz band.
Octurn, Maak's Spirit, and *Aka Moon.*

Name a famous Belgium jazz musician.
Guitarist Philip Catherine and harmonicist Toots Thielemans.

Who was Jean Baptiste "Django" Reinhardt?
The Belgian guitarist who toured America with Duke Ellington's Orchestra and affected the course of American jazz and contemporary music.

Who was Adolphe Sax?
A Belgian musical instrument designer and clarinet musician who invented the saxophone.

Who was Peter Benoit?
A Belgian composer and teacher responsible for the modern revival of Flemish music. In 1867 he founded the Flemish School of Music in Antwerp, which later became the Royal Flemish Conservatory, and served as director until his death.

Who was Cyprien (Cipriano) de Rore?
A Flemish composer who was the first to develop a musical score for voices. His book of madrigals published in the 1500s was the first printed score for voices.

True or false: Originally all musical scores were written for the total orchestra, not individual instruments.
True. Until about 1225, all European music for more than one part was circulated in complete scores, and performers read from these scores.

Who is Sandra Caldarone?
Better known by her stage name Sandra Kim, she is a singer who in 1986 at age 13 became the youngest to win the Eurovision Song Contest.

Who is Helmut Lotti?
A pop singer who became famous by covering Elvis Presley songs.

Who was Henri Vieuxtemps?
A Belgian composer and violinist who began performing at age six. In his later life, after a stroke crippled his use of his arms, he worked to regain the ability to play.

Food

Food in Belgium reflects the many cultures that have mixed and mingled in the country, including the Romans, Vikings, Spanish, French, and English. As a result, a popular saying is that Belgian cooks "cook their food with the finesse of the French but serve it in generous German-size portions!"

Family recipes of hearty stews and soups are handed down from one generation to another. Many tourists come to sample Belgian chocolates and beer and there are festivals for both treats.

A quick snack in Belgium is available at street stands selling waffles and chips. Diners at restaurants are more serious and sit-down meals are seldom hurried.

Belgium is not a country for vegetarians and those with food allergies. For these diners, selections in many parts of the country are very limited.

Recipe

Boeuf carbonnade à la flamande. This recipe from Belgian chef Leon Dhaenens is a popular stew that uses Belgian abbey-style beer. It was modified by Charlie Palmer, chef-owner of *Aureole* in New York City and Las Vegas.

Ingredients.
2 lb. beef chuck, cut into 2" x ½"-thick slices.
Kosher salt and freshly ground black pepper.
1/4 cup flour.
4 Tbsp. unsalted butter.
4 slices bacon, finely chopped.
6 cloves garlic, finely chopped.
3 medium yellow onions, thinly sliced lengthwise.
2 cups Belgian-style ale, such as Ommegang Abbey Ale.
1 cup beef stock.
2 Tbsp. dark brown sugar.
2 Tbsp. apple cider vinegar.
3 sprigs fresh thyme.
3 sprigs fresh parsley.
2 sprigs fresh tarragon.
1 bay leaf.
Bread, for serving.

Preparation. In a bowl, season beef with salt and pepper. Add flour and toss to coat. Heat 2 tablespoons butter in a 6-quart. Dutch oven over medium-high heat. Working in batches, add beef and cook, turning, until browned, about 8 minutes. Transfer to a plate and set aside. Add bacon and cook until the fat renders, about 8 minutes. Add remaining butter and the garlic and onions. Cook until caramelized, about 30 minutes. Add half the beer and cook, scraping bottom of pot, until slightly reduced, about 4 minutes. Return beef to pot with remaining beer, and the stock, sugar, vinegar, thyme, parsley, tarragon, bay leaf, and salt and pepper. Bring to a boil, then reduce heat to medium-low. Cook, covered, until beef is tender, about 1½ hours. Serve with bread.

Food Trivia

True or false: There are over 800 kinds of beers made in Belgium.
True.

How much beer do Belgians consume per year on average?
About 150 liters per person.

Who invented pralines?
Jean Neuhaus in Brussels in 1912.

How much chocolate is produced in Belgium?
About 220,000 tons per year.

What location sells the most chocolate in the world?
Brussels National Airport.

Where were French fries invented?
Belgium.

True or false: Belgium has the most McDonald's restaurants in the world.
False: Belgium has the least per capita in the developed world, seven times less than the United States.

Name three types of Belgian waffles.
Liege waffles are the most common. Brussels waffles are bigger, lighter, rectangular, and eaten with toppings such as strawberries or ice cream. Galettes are thinner, softer, and typically eaten for breakfast, sometimes with jam.

Name a food found in a Belgium bakery.
Cramique is bread made with egg yolks and raisins. Gozettes are turnovers and tarts in flavors including cherry, plum, apple, sugar, and rice.

True or false: The Foire de Libramont is the largest agricultural, forestry and agri-food fair in Europe.
True.

Customs

Weddings

Belgian wedding ceremonies must take place in a local authority's office, such as a city hall of a town where at least one member of the couple is a resident, for the marriage to be legal. The couple may well choose to follow this service with a religious ceremony which takes place after the civil service, usually on the same day.

A Belgian bride carries two flowers down the aisle. Before the ceremony she gives one to her own mother along with a hug. After the wedding ceremony, she presents the other flower to her new mother-in-law and they also embrace, to demonstrate her acceptance into the new family.

During both the civil and religious services there is an exchange of wedding vows and rings. The couple is not permitted to use their own personal vows. The civil service vows include the couple agreeing that each spouse may exert their right to pursue a career without the permission of the other and that their place of residence shall be determined by mutual consent.

At the end of the civil ceremony, the couple is presented with the full text of the marriage law in a little book, which also contains their names, wedding date, and an official city stamp. The book also has space for the couple to write in the names of their children, up to 14 children's names.

Anyone in the general public may attend any civil wedding ceremony. The couple pays for the ceremony, not for the number of guests who attend. Typically, specifically invited guests who attend the civil ceremony then come with the couple to the church service.

Wedding receptions are usually several events with separate guest lists. For example, immediately after the ceremony there may be a champagne reception for all invited guests, so everyone can toast the happy couple's future, but not everyone attends the following formal dinner, which is often only for the couple's immediate family and their closest friends. Traditional Belgian wedding cuisine is seafood, such as cockles, eels, and mussels.

At the sit-down meal, usually husbands and wives are not seated together to encourage everyone to mingle and meet. This reception dinner includes music, dancing, and a special form of cake cutting. After the cutting of the cake, Belgian couples may take part in a custom known as *Le Connemara* during which everyone waves their kerchiefs or napkins in the air and sings.

Children

Although twenty-first century style is to know the birthdate and even pick the name of the child prior to birth, Belgian parents prefer to be surprised and learn the sex of their child at the moment of birth.

It is customary for pregnant women to rub oil on their stomachs to prevent stretch marks and to eat a diet rich in fruit, meat, and dairy.

Traditionally, the child is named for the godparents. However, many modern couples choose a different first name for the child and use a middle name honoring the godparents.

To celebrate the birth, family members gather as soon as possible to see the child and the birth is announced by hanging a stork ornament on the family's front porch.

New mothers spend a full week in the hospital after giving birth. When the new child arrives at home, the family buries the placenta in the yard in thankfulness for new life. On the child's first birthday, the family will plant a tree over the placenta.

Holidays

January 1: New Year's Day.
Date varies: Good Friday.
June 21: Belgium National Day.

November 11: Armistice Day.
December 25: Christmas.
December 31: New Year's Eve.

Customs Trivia

What does a Belgian bride carry on her wedding day?
An heirloom handkerchief embroidered with her name. After the wedding, the handkerchief is framed and hung in the couple's home.

What is the tradition of the wedding handkerchief?
The couple's daughter will receive the handkerchief and her own name will be embroidered on it for her wedding day, and so on through the generations. If the couple doesn't have a daughter, the handkerchief may pass between sisters and through the generations that way, so that it remains an heirloom within the family.

In what language is the civil ceremony performed?
The legal service may be performed in Dutch.

What language is used for the religious wedding ceremony?
Flemish.

True or false: If a guest cannot attend either wedding ceremony, they are still invited to the reception?
True. If a guest is unable to come to either ceremony, they can still be invited to the sit-down meal.

True or false: In Belgium, wedding guests often receive two invitations.
True. It's not uncommon for invitations to be sent out twice, once by the bride's family and again by the groom's to show unity between the families.

What do family members bring to a home to celebrate the birth of a child?
Suikerbonen, a treat made of almonds and chocolate.

Where do family members hang the calendar containing all the birthdays in the family?
In the bathroom.

What happens in the extended family's homes when a new family member is born?
After the announcement of the birth, the new birthday is added to the calendar in the bathroom.

What is the average size of a Belgium family?
Three children.

More Resources

DVDs

Adventures in Europe Volume 1. Destination Amsterdam, DVD. Travel Video Store. Prime Instant Video.

Culinary Travels Discover Belgium, DVD. Vine's Eye Production Inc. Prime Instant Video, 2010.

Gardens of the World. A Japanese Garden in Belgium, DVD. Travel Video Store. Prime Instant Video, 2007.

Globe Trekker: Belgium & Luxembourg, DVD. Pilot Film and TV Productions. Prime Instant Video.

Holland and Belgium, DVD. Queststar, Inc. Prime Instant Video, 2007.

Books

Elliot, M. and H. Smith. *Belgium & Luxembourg Travel Guide* (Lonely Planet, 2013).

Jackson, M. *Great Beers of Belgium* (Brewers Publications, 2008).

Macdonald, M. *Belgium. Culture Smart! a quick guide to customs & etiquette* (Kuperard, 2006).

Steves, R. *Rick Steves' Belgium: Bruges, Brussels, Antwerp, & Ghent* (Avalon Travel Publishing, 2015).

Tait, P., L. McPeake, A. Mason, and D. Colwell. *Eyewitness Travel Guide: Belgium and Luxembourg* (DK Publishing, 2013).

Websites

Map of Belgium: Accessed April 3, 2015,
http://www.worldatlas.com/webimage/countrys/europe/be.htm

Portal Belgium. Accessed April 3, 2015, http://www.belgium.be/en
Tourist Map of Belgium. 2004-2014. Accessed April 3, 2015,
    http://www.eupedia.com/belgium/map_belgium.shtml
US Embassy Belgium. Accessed April 3, 2015,
    http://belgium.usembassy.gov/uspolicy2.html
Visit Belgium Home: Accessed April 3, 2015,
    http://www.visitbelgium.com

Photos

Belgium Photos: Accessed April 3, 2015,
    http://www.trekearth.com/gallery/Europe/Belgium.
Belgium Pictures: Accessed April 3, 2015,
    http://www.planetware.com/pictures/belgium-b.htm.
Belgium: Pictures: Accessed April 3, 2015,
    http://www.tripadvisor.com/LocationPhotos-g188634-Belgium.html
Photos of Belgium: Accessed April 3, 2015,
    http://belgiumphotos.tripod.com
Photos of Belgium: Accessed April 3, 2015,
    http://www.greatbigcanvas.com/category/scenery-by-
    region/europe/belgium/?gclid=CP3g6pen28QCFUZk7AodLGQA5Q

References

Balfolk: Accessed April 3, 2015, http://en.wikipedia.org/wiki/Balfolk
Belgium: Accessed April 3, 2015, http://www.123independenceday.com/belgium/art-
    and-culture.html
Belgium: Accessed March 26, 2015,
    http://www.ask.com/wiki/Geography_of_Belgium?o=2800&qsrc=999&ad=doubleD
    own&an=apn&ap=ask.com
Belgium: Accessed March 27, 2015, http://www.lonelyplanet.com/belgium?affil=ask
Cultural Beliefs of Belgium Mothers: Accessed April 3, 2015,
    http://www.hawcc.hawaii.edu/nursing/RNBelgium10.html
Famous Belgians: Accessed April 3, 2015, http://www.famousbelgians.net/music.htm
Folk Music of Belgium: Accessed April 3, 2015,
    http://www.humanitiesweb.org/human.php?s=g&p=a&a=i&ID=1632
Food Culture in Belgium: Accessed April 3, 2015,
    http://belgium.angloinfo.com/lifestyle/food-and-drink
History of Belgium. 2000–2015. Accessed March 26, 2015,
    http://www.infoplease.com/encyclopedia/world/belgium-history.html

Saveur Carbonnade. Accessed April 3, 2015,
    http://www.saveur.com/article/Recipes/Classic-Beef-Beer-Stew
The 21 Best Luxury Hotels in Belgium. 2015. Accessed March 27, 2015,
    http://www.fivestaralliance.com/luxury-hotels/68/europe/Belgium
Travel Math: Accessed March 27, 2015,
    http://www.travelmath.com/from/Seattle,+WA/to/Brussels,+Belgium
World Wedding Traditions. Belgium Wedding Traditions. Accessed April 3, 2015,
    http://www.worldweddingtraditions.net/belgian-wedding-traditions

DENMARK

Basics

Geography

Denmark is the smallest of the Scandinavian countries and is located on the *Jutland* peninsula, a lowland area. The country also consists of several islands in the Baltic Sea of which the two largest are *Sjælland*, the site of Copenhagen, and *Fyn*. Denmark is about half the size of the US state of Maine.

Language

The official language of the Kingdom of Denmark is Danish. Several minority languages are spoken, including German, Faroese, and Greenlandic. About 86 percent of the population speaks English as a second language.

History

The history of Denmark began with roaming hunters and fisherman communities in about 10,000 to 1500 BC. This population became farmers in Jutland by the end of the eighth century. The population grew to include the Vikings, or Norsemen, who raided Western Europe and the British Isles from the ninth to eleventh centuries

King Harald Blaatand brought Christianity to the country in the tenth century. Harald's son, Sweyn, conquered England in 1013. Sweyn's son, Canute the Great, who reigned from 1014 to 1035, united Denmark, England, and Norway. In fact, the southern tip of Sweden was part of Denmark until the seventeenth century. When Canute died, civil war began and lasted until King Waldemar I reestablished Danish hegemony in the north in 1157. Sweden achieved independence in 1523.

Denmark supported Napoleon and, as a result, in 1815 lost Norway to Sweden. In 1864 the Prussians under Bismarck and the Austrians made war on Denmark as an initial step in the unification of Germany. Denmark was neutral during World War I.

In 1940 Denmark was invaded by the Nazis. King Christian X reluctantly cautioned his fellow Danes to accept the occupation. Denmark was the only occupied country in World War II to save all its Jews from extermination by smuggling them out of the country.

In 1944 Iceland declared its independence from Denmark. In 1948 the Faroe Islands, which had belonged to Denmark since 1380, were granted home rule. In 1953 Greenland officially became a territory of Denmark.

Map and Flag

Flag of Denmark to Color. 2015. Accessed April 4, 2015,
   http://www.coloring.ws/denmark.htm
Map of Denmark. Denmark Coloring Pages. Accessed April 4, 2015,
   http://www.coloring.ws/denmark.htm

Travel

Distance

From New York, NY, to Copenhagen is 3,856 miles. Flight time is 8 hours 13 minutes.

From Chicago, IL, to Copenhagen is 4,263 miles. Flight time is 9 hours 2 minutes.

From Dallas, TX, to Copenhagen is 5,066 miles. Flight time is 10 hours 38 minutes.

From Seattle, WA, to Copenhagen is 4,854 miles. Flight time is 10 hours 13 minutes.

Hotels

Bandholm Hotel. Located in Bandholm, it features a spa, a beach, free breakfast, and an excellent on-site restaurant.

First Hotel Atlantic. Located in Aarhus. Allows pets, has a shared TV/Lounge to allow guests to mingle, and a staff fluent in Dutch, German, English, Norwegian, and Swedish.

Hotel Scandic Webers. Located in Copenhagen. Features 1880s architecture within walking distance of tourist attractions such as *Tivoli*, *Stroget*, and the Round Tower. The hotel also offers bicycles for guests who wish to tour on wheels.

Lillevang. Located in Billund near Legoland. Given a five-star review by all 35 travelers who used Tripadvisor to book this hotel.

Pension Vestergade 44. Located in Aero, it offers free breakfast every morning and its beach has wheelchair access.

Landmarks

Aquadome at Lalandia Billund. Provides a year-round tropical climate with water slides, activity pools, restaurants, shops, entertainment, mini-golf, a bowling center, a sports hall, and a fitness center.

Copenhagen Zoo. Home to more than 3,000 animals of 264 species. The zoo's indoor rainforest houses snakes, crocodiles, marmosets, hornbills, dwarf deer, and free-flying birds and butterflies. In the Children's Zoo guests can see horses being trained.

Legoland. Located in Billund. Home to the world's biggest LEGO™ model, Luke Skywalker's X-wing Starfighter, built from more than 5 million LEGO™ blocks! Visitors can also meet movie characters and watch audiovisual shows.

Louisiana Museum of Modern Art. Located on the North Zealand coast, it features a view across the Sound of Sweden. Its collection of modern art includes international artists such as Jean Arp, Francis Bacon, Alexander Calder, Rene Dubuffet, Max Ernst, Sam Francis, Giacomo Giacometti, Anslem Kiefer, Henry Moore, Pablo Picasso, Robert Rauschenberg, and Andy Warhol.

Tivoli Gardens. Founded in Copenhagen in 1843. Contains beautiful architecture, historic buildings, and lush gardens. At night, thousands of colored lights create an unique fairy-tale atmosphere. Amusement rides, such as the Vertigo, will turn you upside down at 100 km/h — voted Europe's Best Ride in 2014. Tivoli's oldest ride, the wooden roller coaster dating from 1914, is one of only seven roller coasters worldwide which have a brakeman on board every train.

The Blue Planet. Northern Europe's largest aquarium, it features an ocean tank where hammerhead sharks swim together with rays and moray eels in 4 million liters of azure sea water. Guests can see four aquariums from above or below the water level. Three thousand piranhas and anacondas swim under the big waterfall.

Travel Trivia

What does the word *Denmark* mean?
The Land of the Danes.

True or false: It rains every second day in Denmark.
True. The country averages 171 days of precipitation per year.

True or false: There are no islands within Denmark.
False: There are over 100 islands.

True or false: Greenland is the world's largest island.
True.

True or false: Denmark's coastline is longer than the Great Wall of China.
True. It is 7,314 miles in length.

What does the term *LEGO* mean?
It is a combination of the Danish words *leg godt* and means *play well*.

Who created LEGOS™?
Ole Kirk Christiansen started the company in 1932 and produced the first plastic bricks in 1958. There are now 60 LEGO™ blocks for every person on the planet.

True or false: Swimming lessons are mandatory in Denmark.
True.

What breed of dog comes from Denmark?
The Great Dane.

What place in Denmark inspired Disneyland?
Tivoli Gardens.

Who is Janus Frilis?
Creator of the internet telephone company Skype.

What did the US buy from Denmark?
The Virgin Islands in 1917.

What is the legend of the Denmark flag?
The oldest flag in the world, the story goes that it fell from the sky in 1219 during a battle. The Denmark king caught it before it hit the ground and won the battle.

True or false: There are no animals on the Faroe Islands.
False: Sheep outnumber people two to one.

Why did King Christian VII order the construction of Tivoli Gardens?
Legend says the king said, "When people amuse themselves they forget politics."

True or false: Denmark is the world's largest producer of range-raised mink?
True.

Who is Soren Kierkegaard?
A Danish philosopher called the Father of Existentialism.

Who is Karen Blixen?
The author of *Seven Gothic Tales* and *Out of Africa*.

Who is Jens Olsen?
Inventor of the World Clock in Copenhagen. It started keeping time in 1955 and is expected to run for 570,000 years.

What does the word *janteloven* mean?
It is the Danish expression for "You are no better than I am."

America's Roots

Who was Hans Christian Febiger?
Born in Denmark, he came to the American colonies in 1772. He was nicknamed "Old Denmark" and was one of George Washington's most trusted officers during the American Revolution.

Who was Charles Zanco?
A Dane who died at the Alamo in March 1836 during the struggle for Texan independence.

Who was Peter Lassen?
A blacksmith from Copenhagen who led a group of adventurers from Missouri to California in 1839. Lassen is considered one of the most important of California's early settlers and a volcano in northern California, a California county, and a national park bear his name.

Who was Vitus Jonassen Bering?
A Danish explorer who discovered the Bering Strait and was the first European to find Alaska in 1741.

Who was Jens Munk?
A Danish explorer who reached North America in 1619.

Who was Anton Marius Andersen?
An American Lutheran minister and the founding President of Trinity Seminary at Dana College. Born in Denmark, he moved to Wisconsin in 1872.

Who was Victor Borge?
A Danish comedian, conductor, and pianist who achieved great popularity in radio and television in the United States.

Who was Janet Wood Reno?
The first woman to serve as Attorney General of the United States, from 1993 to 2001. She was the second-longest serving Attorney General after William Wirt. Her father was born in Denmark.

Who was Holger Thiele?
An astronomer, actuary, and mathematician, who immigrated to the United States from Denmark, and after whom the asteroid belt body 1586 Thiele is named.

Who is Arthur Charles Nielsen?
He created the TV Nielsen ratings formula. He was born in Chicago and is of Danish descent.

Who is William Webster Hansen?
A US physicist who was one of the founders of the technology of microwave electronics. His father was an immigrant from Denmark.

Who was Jeanette Helen Morrison?
An actress of Danish descent professionally known as Janet Leigh who won a Golden Globe in 1960 for Best Supporting Actress in the movie *Psycho* (1960).

Who was Poul William Anderson?
An American science fiction author who won seven Hugo Awards and three Nebula Awards. Born in Pennsylvania, he lived in Denmark as a child following the death of his father and then returned to the United States in the 1940s.

Who was John Gutzon de la Mothe Borglum?
An American artist and sculptor famous for creating the monumental presidents' heads at Mount Rushmore, South Dakota, the famous carving on Stone Mountain near Atlanta, Georgia, and other public works of art, including a bust of Abraham Lincoln which was exhibited in Theodore Roosevelt's White House and then kept in the crypt of the United States Capitol in Washington, DC. He was the son of Danish Immigrants.

Who was Jens Christen Clausen?
A Danish-American botanist, geneticist, and ecologist. He is considered a pioneer in the field of ecological and evolutionary plant genetics.

Sports and Games

Sports

Sports are an important part of Danish culture. Three out of four children and about half of the adult population participate in sports on a regular basis.

Two million out of a population of 5.5 million Danes are members of at least one of Denmark's more than 14,000 sports associations. The clubs began in rural societies over a century ago and arrived in the large cities during the early twentieth century. The Danish sports club model is built on voluntary work, openness, and joint responsibility. Club coaches and sport officials often are volunteers.

As in most of Europe, football, which Americans call soccer, is the most popular sport in Denmark, with over 300,000 players and 1,614 clubs registered with the Danish Football Association.

There are four professional football leagues which include 60 of the best clubs in Denmark. The national Danish women's football team has competed in nine World Cups and 11 European Championships. The team won the European Championship in 1979.

Handball is the second-most popular sport and the most popular during the winter. The national handball association has over 160,000 male and female members. Other popular sports include cycling, sailing sports, badminton, ice hockey, swimming, and, a recent addition, golf. And there is a growing interest in American basketball.

Sports Trivia

When was the Danish Football Association *Dansk Boldspil-Union* founded?
1889.

True or false: The national Danish men's football team won two Olympic silver medals in 1908 and 1912 and was ranked number one in the world between April 1914 and April 1920.
True.

True or false: In 1978, the men's football league turned professional with the first sponsor being Carlsberg Brewery.
True.

What is the name of the largest football stadium in Denmark?
Parken, which has 38,009 seats.

Who is a *roligan*?
A traveling fan. The objectives of the *roligan* movement were to remain calm yet cheerful and be supportive during matches. *Rolig* means *calm* in the Danish language.

True or false: Handball was invented by the Danes.
True.

Who is Bjarne Riis?
The only Dane to win the Tour de France.

What was Copenhagen originally?
A fishing colony.

True or false: Denmark is Europe´s strongest badminton country.
True. The country has won 10 gold medals since the start of the World Championships in 1977.

Who is Poul-Erik Høyer Larsen?
The winner of the 1996 Olympic Games gold medal in badminton.

Game

Kick the Kitty Cat. This traditional game is based on putting a live cat inside a barrel. But don't worry — the cruel part of the game no longer exists, and a fun, modified tradition has survived.

Number of players. Ten.

Materials. A wooden barrel, candy and small prizes, a hook, wooden sticks, and a rope. Modified for residents: Inflate a very large balloon and tie off the end. Cover the surface of the balloon completely in string except for a 2" by 2" square. Paint the string with glue. When the glue dries, pop and remove the balloon. Now fill the empty string balloon with candy and tape the opening shut.

To play. Resident players take turns rolling and shaking the balloon until it breaks open.

Winner. Everybody who participates gets a share of the loot, but there are two winners in the game: the Cat Queen, the person who breaks the barrel/balloon, and the Cat King, the person who knocks down the last remaining part of the barrel/balloon.

ICHI benefits. Mental function of language, articulation, mobility of joints, muscle force, and control of voluntary movements.

Music and Dance

Music

Music is so important in Denmark that during special celebrations such as birthdays, weddings, and anniversaries not only is music played but it is customary for guests to write songs for those being celebrated.

There are many choirs throughout the country which specialize in traditional Danish songs or folk music. The Danish Folk Council promotes folk music around the world. There are over 12,000 folk dancers belonging to more than 200 local clubs in Denmark.

Traditional folk music is played on fiddles and accordions. Danish fiddlers usually play in groups. Fiddle and accordion duos play the rhythmic Nordic folk dance music. The oldest variety of this music is called *pol* and has been played for more than 170 years.

The *lur* is a wind instrument and the national symbol of Denmark. This long horn has no finger holes. It can be straight or curved in various shapes, and can be made of bronze or wood.

Until around 1900, traditional music was the common musical culture of Denmark, but classical music spread and folk music remained popular only in rural areas.

Music Videos

Danish String Quartet Plays Sonderho Bridal Trilogy: Accessed April 4, 2015, https://www.youtube.com/watch?v=6Ey_tNIAmRU

Danish String Quartet Plays *Wood Works*: Accessed April 4, 2015, https://www.youtube.com/watch?v=ZTH6VxQwZLM

Faroe Islands Folk Music Festival Mykines: Accessed January 17, 2016, https://m.youtube.com/watch+G221g7ScVI4

Viking Instrument Lur: Accessed January 17, 2016, https://m.youtube.com/watch?v=wsAHiiY7Rc0

Viking Tones #1 Lur-calls: Accessed January 17, 2016, https://www.youtube.com/watch?v=DRSVcOHlLP8

Dance

In the early history of Denmark, music called *spillemandsmusik* was common and most towns had one or more town musicians to play for dances, processions, and certain rituals. In the seventeenth and eighteenth centuries, professional music performances were monopolized by these town musicians, who also traveled into the neighboring rural areas to perform. Also during that time, the fiddle was introduced and became the most important instrument, and chain dances were replaced by pair dances.

At the end of the eighteenth century, English-style contra and square dances became popular. During the nineteenth century the waltz became the most popular dance in the cities, after having first been danced in the countryside. Around 1850 the polka and mazurka were popular repertoire but by the end of the nineteenth century, earlier dance traditions were replaced with dances from England, Southern Europe, and America.

The Association for the Promotion of Folkdancing was founded in 1901 with the goal to preserve popular dances from the period 1750 to 1850.

Dance Videos

Barn Dance Denmark Molposen "The Moth Bag": Accessed January 17, 2016, https://m.youtube.com/watch?v=ntB48fW7U9o

Danish Folk Dance — Masquerade: Accessed April 4, 2015, https://www.youtube.com/watch?v=Ch_LweerOQQ

Danish Traditional Dance at Solvang: Accessed January 17, 2016, https://m.youtube.com/watch?v=xzH4YGoNHf4

Folk Dance in Denmark Seven Jumps: Accessed January 17, 2016, https://m.youtube.com/watch?v=SUn5GI9cPtk

Folk Dance in Denmark Part 1: Accessed January 17, 2016, https://m.youtube.com/watch?v=gcTl-c4gWPM

Music and Dance Trivia

True or false: Denmark has two national anthems.
True. *Der er et Yndigt Land*, meaning *there is a lovely land* is more common and is sung at sporting events. *Kong Kristian Stod ved Højen*

Mast, meaning *King Christian stood by towering mast,* is used on official occasions when the royal family is present.

Why did drums, bagpipes, and hurdy-gurdies fade out of folk music?
During the seventeenth century these instruments were considered improper for making music.

What is the most popular instrument for folk dancing?
The fiddle.

What is a chain dance?
A ceremonial dance accompanied by pipes, drums, and singing.

Who was Rasmus Storm?
A folk musician from the 1700s.

Who was Svend Grundtvig?
A folk musician in the 1800s.

Who was A. P. Berggreen?
A music publisher in the 1800s.

Who was Evald Tang Kristensen?
He published Denmark songs in the early twentieth century.

What is ethnology?
The study and collection of folk tradition including music, song, and dances.

What area of the country kept folk music and dance alive into the twenty-first century?
Jutland.

Food

Most people in Denmark eat at home and bring their lunches to work. Breakfast is usually coffee or tea and rye bread or white bread with cheese or jam for adults, and cereals with milk for children. The traditional morning meal of *junket crumble,* a mixture of grated rye bread and brown sugar, or *ollebrod,* a dish made of rye bread, sugar, and non-alcoholic beer, have been eaten for breakfast since the middle ages but is no longer the norm.

Starting in the nineteenth century, special kinds of breakfast bread — small round, flat, or crescent-shaped wheat rolls — became popular. These are eaten only in the morning and are available at shops throughout the country. Breakfast on Sunday is usually breakfast rolls with cheese or jam and *wienerbrod* — flaky pastries made of rich bread dough rolled out several times in layers with butter between and filled with custard or a mixture of butter, sugar, and cinnamon. In addition, fruit juice is often served and sometimes a glass of *Gammel Dansk* or another bitter.

Lunch is usually a cold meal consisting of slices of rye bread buttered and covered with various kinds of sausage, sliced boiled egg, or liver paste, a baked and spreadable mixture of chopped pig's liver and lard. A traditional open-faced sandwich for lunch can be made of any of the following: cold fish, fried fish, pickles, mayonnaise, cold meats, tartar, roast beef, smoked sausage, chicken salad, eggs, and occasionally a combination of vegetables such as potato, onion, and tomato.

Most Danes make an effort to gather the family around a hot meal every evening. Traditionally this was gruel, meat broth, or sweet fruit soup followed by a main course of meat or fish and, always, potatoes and gravy. Even today, Danes eat mainly minced meats and meat cuts for pan-frying along with traditional gravy and potato dishes.

Recipe

Walnut Cake. Usually baked three days before serving and topped with whipped cream when served. In small slices, this can serve 20.

Ingredients.

8 ounces unsalted butter

6 tablespoons raw sugar

7 cups walnut halves

¾ cup all-purpose flour

1½ cup almond flour or almond meal

¾ cup granulated sugar

6 large eggs

¾ cup heavy cream

½ cup plain whole-milk yogurt

1 tsp. salt

1 vanilla bean, split lengthwise

Whipped cream

Preparation. Preheat the oven to 350 degrees F. Butter a metal or glass baking dish. Sprinkle the bottom evenly with 3 tablespoons of raw sugar and set aside. Coarsely chop the walnuts in a food processor and set 2 cups aside. Add all-purpose flour to the processor and pulse until the walnuts are very finely ground, about 1–2 minutes. Add almond flour. Pulse to blend and set aside.

Using an electric mixer, in a large bowl beat the butter and granulated sugar until light and fluffy. Add eggs, cream, yogurt, and salt, and scrape in the seeds from the vanilla bean. Beat until well combined. Add ground-walnut mixture and beat just to blend. Gently fold in the chopped walnuts, while being careful not to overmix. Pour batter into prepared dish and smooth top. Sprinkle with remaining 3 tablespoons raw sugar. Bake for 50 to 55 minutes.

Food Trivia

What is served to guests at breakfast for special occasions, such as birthdays and anniversaries?
Wienerbrod.

True or false: Denmark invented the brunch.
False: The American brunch was introduced in the late twentieth century.

What is a warm meat served at lunch?
Roasted sausages.

What sweet is served in the winter?
Apple cakes.

What sweet is served in the summer?
Strawberry soup.

What dessert is served in the spring?
Rhubarb trifle.

Why does the wait staff in a Denmark restaurant not write down the food orders?
Legend says that when the army officers' association dined at Tivoli, the restaurant staff introduced a list of the many varieties and combinations of ingredients which the officers could use to write their own open-faced

sandwich requests as remembering or writing orders was too hard for the busy wait staff.

How did the open-faced sandwich become a lunch favorite?
Legend says that in the sixteenth century slices of bread were used instead of plates because plates were expensive and rare.

Why is dinner called *middag*?
Dinner used to be eaten in the middle of the day.

What is the traditional first course in a Sunday evening meal?
Pudding.

Customs

Weddings

In most of the world, traditionally the man proposes to the woman but in Denmark the couple buys the wedding rings together and share the cost. The preparation and cost of the wedding is also shared between the bride and groom, not the bride's parents, as in America. The groom also purchases the bridal bouquet.

As in America, the white wedding dress is bought by the bride and is not to be seen by the groom before the wedding. The bride needs to wear four things: something new, old, borrowed, and blue — and guests may demand to see all four.

In Denmark most couples live together for several years before they get married, but the night before the wedding the bride and groom are supposed to sleep separately. On the wedding day the groom arrives at the church 30 minutes before the wedding and the bride arrives 5 minutes before and is escorted by her father. Some couples marry in civil ceremonies at the town hall.

After the wedding ceremony the couple is greeted outside by friends throwing rice. Danish weddings are typically kept quite small with only close family and friends attending, so on average there are 25 to 80 guests.

The ceremony is followed by photos and a dinner with speeches, songs, fun games, and dancing. There is a special order in which to conduct the speeches: first the bride's father, then the groom, followed by the bride, then family members, and finally, friends.

Children

Most births are monitored in the hospital by a midwife without a doctor present. A woman may also choose a home birth. Giving birth into water in a home or hospital birthing pool is becoming popular.

After the birth, mother and infant stay in the maternity ward for two to three hours and then move to another room where advice is provided about care of the newborn and breast feeding. Most mothers in Denmark breastfeed for at least six months.

During the first year of the child's life, a nurse makes home visits to ensure mother and baby are well, monitor baby's health, and offer advice. The first visit from the health visitor occurs a week after the birth. Subsequent visits usually take place every quarter.

All births are recorded by the Registrar of the State Church who issues a birth certificate. The birth forms completed by a midwife must be handed in at the local State Church office in the area of residence within 14 days of the birth, even if the family are affiliated with another religion or do not attend church.

The child must have at least one Danish National as a parent to become a Danish citizen. Parents have up to six months after the birth to choose the surname of their child born in Denmark. The name must be permitted under the Danish Act on Names. Parents who are or have been foreign nationals are allowed to give their child a surname that is not approved in Denmark as long as the name is approved in the parents' home country.

Holidays

January 1: New Year's Day.
Variable date: Good Friday.
Variable date: Easter.
Variable date: Easter Monday.
Variable date: Whit Monday, the day after Pentecost.
Variable date: Ascension Day.
June 5: Constitution Day.

December 25: Christmas.
December 31: New Year's Eve.

Customs Trivia

What do guests do when the bride or groom leaves the reception room?
Kiss the spouse who remains.

Why do guests bang on plates and glasses during the dinner?
To request the bride and groom to sit and kiss.

Why must the wedding waltz be danced before midnight?
To ensure good luck throughout the marriage.

What must male friends do for the groom at the reception?
Lift the groom up and cut off the tip of his socks. This symbolizes that now he should no longer walk in the footsteps of other women.

How does the wedding reception end?
With dancing and drinking toasts.

What is *Fastelavn*?
The celebration before the start of Lent, similar to Halloween in the United States. Children wear a costume and go door-to-door seeking candy or money.

What do children sing at each door during Fastelavn?
"Yummy, yummy, yummy, sweet buns in my tummy."

What is a *Fastelavnsboller*?
A sweet bun that children are given during Fastelavn.

What is a *fastelavnsris*?
A bunch of birch branches decorated with small paper shapes and pieces of candy which is given to children during Fastelavn.

How much childcare leave do new parents receive?
The mother receives six months but she can give the last three months to the father.

More Resources

DVDs

Global Treasures Copenhagen Kobenhavn Denmark. Travel Video Store. Prime Instant Video, 2009.

Global Treasures Rosenborg Castle Rosenborg Slot Kobenhavn Denmark. NR CC Travel Video Store. Prime Instant Video.

Globe Trekker. Sweden & Denmark. Pilot Film and Television Productions. Ltd. Prime Instant Video, 2006.

Solvang: A Little Bit of Denmark. Travel Video Store. Prime Instant Video, 2009.

Vista Point Copenhagen Denmark. Travel Video Store. Prime Instant Video, 2007.

Books

Bain, C., C. Bonetto, and A. Stone. *Lonely Planet Denmark* (Lonely Planet, 2012).

Cunningham, A., Plumer, J. Spaull, and L. Mouritsen. 2013. *Top 10 Copenhagen* (DK Travel; 2013).

DK Eyewitness Travel Guide, *Denmark Paperback* (DK Publishing, 2013).

Mouritsen, L. and R. Norum. *Pocket Rough Guide Copenhagen* (Rough Guides, 2014).

Steves, R. *Rick Steves' Snapshot Copenhagen & the Best of Denmark* (Avalon Travel Publishing, 2012).

Websites

Denmark. The official website of Denmark: Accessed April 4, 2015, http://denmark.dk/en/society/government-and-politics

Flag of Denmark: Accessed April 4, 2015, http://www.mapsofworld.com/flags/denmark-flag.html

United States Website on Denmark: Accessed April 4, 2015, http://denmark.usembassy.gov/visa/escams.html

Visit Denmark. The official website for tourists: Accessed April 4, 2015, http://www.visitdenmark.com/denmark/tourist-frontpage

Photos

Copenhagen Pictures: Accessed April 4, 2015,
  http://www.copenhagenpictures.dk

Denmark: Accessed April 4, 2015, http://www.earth-
  photography.com/Countries/Denmark

Denmark Pictures and Images: Accessed April 4, 2015,
  http://photobucket.com/images/denmark

Photo Gallery: Denmark's Castle Country: Accessed April 4, 2015,
  http://travel.nationalgeographic.com/travel/countries/denmark-castle-
  country-photos-traveler

Photos of Denmark: Accessed April 4, 2015,
  http://www.tripadvisor.com/LocationPhotos-g189512-Denmark.html

References

68 Interesting Facts about Denmark: Accessed April 4, 2015,
  http://facts.randomhistory.com/denmark-facts.html

Copenhagen: Accessed April 4, 2015,
  http://www.travelmath.com/from/Seattle,+WA/to/Copenhagen,+Denmark

Danish Americans: Accessed April 4, 2015, http://www.everyculture.com/multi/Bu-
  Dr/Danish-Americans.html

Danish Folk Music and Instruments: Accessed April 4, 2015,
  http://dinolingo.com/blog/2013/09/17/danish-folk-music-and-instruments-danish-
  culture-for-kids/#.VR_gF5M__e4

Danish Traditional Music: Accessed April 4, 2015,
  http://en.wikipedia.org/wiki/Danish_traditional_music

Denmark: Accessed April 4, 2015,
  http://www.infoplease.com/country/denmark.html?pageno=5

Denmark Coloring Pages: Accessed April 4, 2015, http://www.coloring.ws/denmark.htm

Denmark. New Nordic Recipes. Walnut Cake: Accessed April 4, 2015,
  http://denmark.dk/en/lifestyle/food-drink/new-nordic-recipes

Having a Baby in Denmark: Accessed April 4, 2015,
  http://denmark.angloinfo.com/healthcare/pregnancy-birth

Hotels in Denmark: Accessed April 4, 2015, http://www.tripadvisor.com/Hotel_Review-
  g2555876-d2071815-Reviews-Bandholm_Hotel-
  Bandholm_Lolland_Municipality_Lolland_South_Zealand_Zealand.html

Languages of Denmark: Accessed April 4, 2015,
  http://www.ask.com/wiki/Languages_of_Denmark?o=2800&qsrc=999&ad=double
  Down&an=apn&ap=ask.com

Notable Danish Americans: Accessed January 17, 2016,
  https://en.m.wikipedia.org/wiki/Danish_Americans

Sport, the Official Website of Denmark: Accessed April 4, 2015,
    http://denmark.dk/en/lifestyle/sport

The Natives. Meet the Kids: Accessed April 4, 2015,
    http://kids.denmark.dk/Traditions_eng.htm

Traditional Danish Wedding with All the Customs, Beauty, and Fun: Accessed April 4,
    2015, http://www.earthoria.com/traditional-danish-wedding-with-all-the-customs-
    beauty-and-fun.html

Visit Denmark: http://www.visitdenmark.com/guide/denmarks-most-visited-attractions

ENGLAND

Basics

Geography

The United Kingdom of Great Britain and Northern Ireland includes the areas of England in the south, Scotland in the north, and Wales in the west. It includes land on two islands, the northern one-sixth of the island of Ireland and all of the island of the United Kingdom. It is located in Western Europe between the North Atlantic Ocean and the North Sea, northwest of France. There are also about 100 smaller islands in the North and Irish Seas and English Channel that fall within the boundaries of the country. This chapter looks at the part that is England.

England is a country of gently rolling hills and lowlands with several large rivers. The Thames River, the longest in the country, runs through London. England itself is the largest region of the United Kingdom with a population of over 51 million people (2008). England is 74 times smaller than the United States.

Language

The official language is English. Recent immigrants from Pakistan have introduced Punjabi and Urdu into the country.

History

Historians believe that humans lived on the land now called England about 8,000 years ago. The Celts arrived from Europe around 1,000 BC. The Romans invaded the island in 55 BC and in 43 AD, when they began their rule of the country that lasted for 400 years. During the last 100 years of this period, the original inhabitants revolted. Beginning in 410 AD, the Romans left England.

After the Romans, there was fighting between tribes and communities throughout the country. An Anglo-Saxon establishment in Kent in 455 AD was the beginning of a unified country. In 601 AD written laws were established.

Over the next several centuries, Norway and France invaded England, and there was more fighting between areas of today's Wales, Scotland, and England. King Henry I came to power in 1100, formed treaties with France and other neighboring countries, and also established a system of laws — which he himself violated.

The medieval period found more fighting for territory by a series of kings. King Henry VIII took the throne in 1509. The Union Jack, the nation's flag, was established in 1607.

The British Empire started to grow and in 1713 included Nova Scotia, Newfoundland, Minorca, Gibraltar, and the American colonies, as well as the sole right to supply slaves to Spanish colonies. Cornwallis surrendered his British troops at Yorktown, and the treaty ending the war with the American colonies was signed on September 3, 1783. At one time, the saying "The sun never sets on the British Empire" was true as the country's colonies included India and Hong Kong, but over time these were lost in battle and surrendered in treaty.

Today's United Kingdom countries are England, Wales, Scotland, and Northern Ireland.

Map and Flag

British Isles Printout: Accessed March 8, 2015,
   http://www.enchantedlearning.com/europe/britain/flag.shtml
Flag of the United Kingdom: Accessed March 8, 2015,
   http://www.enchantedlearning.com/europe/britain/flag.shtml

Travel

Distance

From New York, NY, to London, England is 3,471 miles. Flight time is 7 hours 27 minutes.

From Chicago, IL, to London, England is 3,959 miles. Flight time is 8 hours 25 minutes.

From Dallas, TX, to London, England is 4,759 miles. Flight time is 10 hours 1 minute.

From Seattle, WA, to London, England is 4,799 miles. Flight time is 10 hours 6 minutes.

Hotels

Egerton House Hotel. Located at 17-19 Egerton Terrace in Knightsbridge, London. Winner of the 2015 Traveler's Choice Award for luxury. Offers free breakfast every morning and is 0.2 miles from the Victoria and Albert Museum.

St. Ermin's Hotel. Located on Caxton Street in Westminster, London, near St. James's Park, Parliament Square, the London Eye, Westminster Abbey, and Houses of Parliament. Allows pets.

The Goring Beeston Place. Located in Grosvenor Gardens, London. Provides shuttle bus service and is located 0.8 miles from the world-famous Harrods department store.

The Royal Horseguards Hotel. Located at 2 Whitehall Court, London. Has a fitness center and is located 0.2 miles from the Horse Guards Parade at Whitehall.

The Rubens at the Palace. Located at 39 Buckingham Palace Road in Victoria, London. Has a tennis court and is 0.2 miles from Buckingham Palace.

Landmarks

Buckingham Palace. This 600-room palace is the home of the royal family and is surrounded by a 40 acre garden.

Kings College. Founded in 1441 by King Henry VI. A part of the University of Cambridge.

Mother Shipton's Cave. Near Knaresborough, North Yorkshire. England's oldest recorded tourist attraction. In 1630 its owner Charles Slingsby fenced off the site and started charging visitors to view its petrifying well. The mineral-rich water from the spring has the ability to give objects a stone-like appearance after a prolonged exposure.

Stonehenge. Located on Salisbury Plain southwest of London. A prehistoric monument dating back over 5,000 years. This circle of stone monuments is a mystery to archaeologists and may have been built as a worship site or market place.

Tower of London. Built next to the Thames River by William the Conqueror in 1066. The location of many famous executions and imprisonments including Anne Boleyn, Catherine Howard, Lady Jane Gray, and Sir Walter Raleigh. The tower is also home of the Crown Jewels.

Windsor Castle. The home of the royal family for over 900 years. The royal flag is flown over the castle only when the king or queen is in residence. Built by the Normans. Located by the Thames River.

Travel Trivia

Who was Sir Walter Raleigh?
The Englishman who planted the first potatoes in Ireland in the 1600s. In 1592 Raleigh was given many rewards by the Queen, including Durham House in the Strand and the estate of Sherborne, Dorset. However, he was beheaded at Whitehall on October 29, 1618.

Who was Sir Francis Drake?
He led the first English circumnavigation of the world, from 1577 to 1580. On September 26, 1580, his ship *The Golden Hind* sailed into Plymouth with Drake and 59 remaining crew aboard, along with a rich cargo of spices and captured Spanish treasures. Drakes Bay, which many believe was his first landing place in California, is named for him.

Who was Captain James Cook?
An Englishman who was the first to map Newfoundland, prior to making three voyages to the Pacific Ocean during which he achieved the first European contact with the eastern coastline of Australia and the Hawaiian Islands as well as the first recorded circumnavigation of New

Zealand. This led to the establishment of an English penal colony and gradual non-native settlement of Australia.

Who was William Shakespeare?

A playwright and poet whose work is considered the greatest in English literature. He wrote dozens of plays which continue to dominate world theater 400 years later.

Who was Sir Isaac Newton?

A mathematician and scientist who invented differential calculus and formulated the theory of universal gravitation, the nature of light, and the three laws of motion. He is considered the smartest man who ever lived.

True or false: Most of America's founding fathers have a common ancestry.

True. The majority of the Founding Fathers of the United States of America were of English extraction, including Benjamin Franklin, George Washington, John Adams, James Madison, and Thomas Jefferson.

Who is Isambard Kingdom Brunel?

A famous engineer of Victorian times.

What happens if two women pour from the same teapot?

They will quarrel.

What church in London has the second largest dome in the world?

St. Paul's Cathedral is second only to St. Peter's in Rome, Italy.

When was the Great Fire of London?

September 2, 1666. It destroyed a large area of the city including St. Paul's. It took 35 years to rebuild to the church.

Who was Jack the Ripper?

A serial killer who murdered at least five people in London in the late nineteenth century and never was caught.

What musical group started the British Invasion of America?

The Beatles: Paul McCartney, John Lennon, George Harrison, and Ringo Starr.

What is Blackpool Tower?

A famous seaside landmark in Lancashire opened to the public in 1894.

What is the London Eye?
A Ferris wheel in London that stands 450 feet tall and can carry 800 passengers on a 30-minute ride.

Who was Charles Dickens?
A Victorian writer of *A Christmas Carol* and other English novels.

What is the hottest temperature ever recorded in England?
101.3 degrees F. in Brogdale, Kent, in August 2003.

True or false: English people drink the most tea in the world.
True. They consume more tea per capita than anybody else in the world, 22 times more than Americans.

True or false: Among the three ghosts said to haunt Athelhampton House is an ape.
True.

Where is the world's most diverse wildfowl center?
The Slimbridge Wildlife and Wetlands Trust is the world's largest and most diversified wildfowl center. It has the largest collection of swans, geese, and ducks on Earth, and is the only place where all six species of flamingo can still be observed.

America's Roots

Who was Virginia Dare?
The first English child born in the Thirteen Colonies, in 1587, to English parents at Roanoke Island in what is present-day North Carolina.

Who was Lucille Ball?
A comedian; a film, television, stage, and radio actress; a model; a film and television executive. She became the first woman to run a major television studio, Desilu, which produced many successful and popular television series. She won four Emmy Awards, the Women in Film Crystal Award, the Golden Globe Cecil B. DeMille Award, the Kennedy Center Honors Lifetime Achievement Award, and the Academy of Television Arts & Sciences Governors' Award. She was of English descent.

Who is Hillary Diane Rodham Clinton?

She was the sixty-seventh US Secretary of State, serving in the administration of President Barack Obama. She was a United States Senator for New York from 2001 to 2009. She is the wife of the forty-second US President. She is of English descent.

Who was Ulysses S. Grant?

The eighteenth US President and the Union general who led the defeat of the Confederate military. He was of English descent.

Who was Robert Edward Lee?

He commanded the Confederate Army during the American Civil War and was the son of Revolutionary War officer Henry "Light Horse Harry" Lee III.

Who is David Letterman?

A recently retired late-night talk-show host and comedian of English descent.

Who is Robert De Niro?

Critics believe he is one of the greatest American actors of all time. His ancestry is Italian, Irish, German, Dutch, English, and French.

Who is Cameron Diaz?

An American actress whose mother is of English, Scots-Irish, and German ancestry.

Who is Chevy Chase?

An American comedian and actor whose ancestors came from England.

Who is John Glenn?

An American astronaut, the first American to orbit the Earth, and the fifth person in space. He flew on the Friendship Seven. His ancestors are from England.

Who is Alan Bartlett "Al" Shepard, Jr.?

One of the original NASA Mercury Seven astronauts who in 1961 became the second person and the first American to travel into space. He was also the fifth and oldest person to walk on the moon. His ancestors are from England.

Who was Percival Lawrence Lowell?

An astronomer of English descent who founded the Lowell Observatory in Flagstaff, Arizona, and began the work that led to the discovery of Pluto 14 years after his death.

Who was Wyatt Berry Stapp Earp?

A deputy town marshal in Tombstone, Arizona, who took part in the gunfight at the OK Corral during which lawmen killed three outlaw cowboys. His ancestors were from England.

Who is James Danforth "Dan" Quayle?

He was the forty-fourth Vice President of the United States under President George H. W. Bush. His great-great grandfather was born in England.

Who was Henry Chadwick?

An English-born American sportswriter, baseball statistician, and historian, often called "the father of baseball" for his early reporting on and contributions to the development of the game. He edited the first baseball guide that was sold to the public. He is credited with creating box scores, as well as creating the abbreviation *K* that designates a strikeout.

Sports and Games

Sports

When it comes to sports in England as well as in the United Kingdom, football, which Americans call soccer, is the most popular game. There are more than 100 teams. The 20 most elite teams, chosen from all over the United Kingdom, form the premier league, of which the most famous are Manchester United, Liverpool, and Arsenal. Football in the United Kingdom is backed by a governing body known as the Football Association, which is one of the oldest football-governing bodies in the world. The Football Association (FA) Cup and the Capital One Cup are the two of the most famous football championships in the United Kingdom. Ninety-two professional football clubs participate under four main divisions in each of these tournaments each year.

Cricket is the national game of the United Kingdom. The sport began in England and spread to hundreds of countries around the world. During the eighteenth century, when cricket started and then grew in popularity very rapidly all over the world, researchers and players met at Marylebone Cricket Club (MCC) on Lord's Cricket ground to finalize cricket rules. There are more than 20 cricket clubs in the United Kingdom and there are thousands of cricket teams in the country. The first-class UK country championship is the oldest cricket championship in the world.

Rugby, a very popular sport in England, was originally played only by the elite, but now is a game for the masses.

The Badminton Association of England was established in 1893 and today provides league and club structure in England.

The first English tennis was played in London around 1877. Today Wimbledon is one of the four Grand Slam tennis tournaments. The other three are the Australian Open, the US Open, and the French Open.

Additional popular sports include swimming, rowing, ice hockey, and netball.

Sports Trivia

What is worm-charming?
An English sport in which each competitor has to gather as many worms as possible from a 3-meter x 3-meter plot of land in a set time. No digging or use of liquids of any kind is allowed.

Who is the world champion bog snorkler?
Joanne Pitchforth, with a time of 1 minute 35 seconds.

What is bog-snorkling?
Originating in Llanwrtyd Wells in 1985, it has become an annual contest attracting competitors from all over the world. A 60-yard trench is cut through a peat bog and contestants must negotiate two lengths wearing snorkels and flippers. Wetsuits are usually worn but die-hard bog-snorklers scorn such frippery.

What is cheese rolling?
A 200 year old game in which a large, round Double-Gloucester cheese is set rolling at the top of a steep hill and a group of competitors must run

after it and try to catch it. The cheese is rarely caught as it is estimated it can reach speeds approaching 70 mph.

What sport was created in England in 1954?

Underwater hockey, also known as *octopush*, was first created by Alan Blake of Southsea Sub-Aqua Club. Most of the action takes place on the floor of a swimming pool and competitors wear snorkels.

What sport was created in an English pub in 1974?

Lawn mower racing.

What is Welly-wanging?

The sport of throwing a Wellington boot as far as possible which probably started in Yorkshire. The goal is to get maximum speed through the shoulder and down the forearm to the Welly.

Who is Phil Shaw?

The creator of the sport of extreme ironing.

What is extreme ironing?

The story goes that Phil Shaw came home from work one evening and the thought of ironing didn't appeal, even though it had to be done. He would much rather have been out rock-climbing so, being a practical sort of chap, he decided to combine the two, and the sport of extreme ironing was born. He promoted the activity using the alias *Steam*. Extreme ironing has become popular in countries as widespread as Germany and New Zealand. Followers have performed extreme ironing on top of mountains, on top of famous landmarks, down river rapids, under the sea, and even while bungee-jumping.

What is the game Sack of Wool?

Players race while carrying a heavy sack of wool, around 60 pounds, along a 280-yard course with uphill gradients of around 1 in 4. The race has been in existence for many hundreds of years and originated from local men trying to impress the girls at the end of a day of sheepshearing. Today there are also female competitions.

Game

Old Maid. This card game, well known to American children, originated in nineteenth century England where it was based on a drinking game. While there are specially made Old Maid cards, the game can be played with a regular deck by removing one of the queens.

Number of players. Six.

Materials. A deck of Old Maid cards or a deck of 52 standard cards with one queen removed.

To play. Players take turns selecting a random card from the player to their right. If they can make a pair, they discard that pair. The game continues until one player is left holding the spare queen, called the "old maid."

Winner. The player holding the spare queen loses.

ICHI benefits. Mental functions of language, speech, control of voluntary movement, muscle force, and mobility of joints.

Music and Dance

Music

Indigenous folk music has survived for thousands of years in England and has become popular pub music for the past 40 years. One example is *Greensleeves* which is believed to have been written by King Henry VIII for Queen Anne Boleyn. It has the same melody as the Christmas hymn *What Child is This?*

The chorus is familiar:

Greensleeves was all my joy,
Greensleeves was my delight,
Greensleeves was my heart of gold,
And who but my Lady Greensleeves.

English music took worldwide center stage in the 1960s with what Americans call the British Invasion. The Beatles appeared on the US TV show *Ed Sullivan* and American teenagers fell madly in love with the band members and their sound. The group topped the charts with six of the top ten albums and 21 of the top singles of the decade. They were followed by the Rolling Stones, Elton John, Herman's Hermits, and more.

In the 1970s, England gave the world Andrew Lloyd Weber who created musicals *Jesus Christ Superstar*, *Cats*, *Phantom of the Opera*, and many more.

Music Videos

Beatles. Love Me Do: Accessed January 17, 2016,
  https://m.youtube.com/watch?v=yAmkNDX3GRU
Elton John at the Royal Opera House: Accessed January 17, 2016,
  https://m.youtube.com/watch?v=vschhZ7TxlM
Greensleeves: Accessed January 17, 2016,
  https://m.youtube.com/watch?v=twix9KfES9Y

Dance

English country dance began in the sixteenth century and is a mixture of folk dance and dance styles from Europe. A popular folk dance still in fashion is the May Pole dance which is performed around a pole with ribbons intertwined by the dancers. As the dancers move in a circle around the pole, they weave in and out, thus wrapping the pole with ribbons. The dance dates back over 2000 years to Rome's occupation of what is now England, when a festival honored Flora, the Roman goddess of fruit and flowers. Today the dance is performed on the first day of May to celebrate the coming of warmer weather.

Dancing was popular in the court of the king, thus dance masters would create new dances to win approval from the monarch.

Throughout the seventeenth century, country dancing was popular throughout England, Scotland, Ireland, Europe, and the American colonies. During the eighteenth century, public ballrooms, such as the Assembly Rooms at Bath, made country dancing available to the general public. It reached a peak of popularity in the eighteenth century and then faded with the rise of waltz, polka, and other couples dances in the early nineteenth century.

Cecil Sharp, an English musicologist and teacher, re-interpreted country dances for contemporary audiences in the mid-nineteenth century. Through his hard work, interest in these dances continued to grow in the twentieth century and new dances and tunes in English country dance style have been composed by English, American, and European composers.

Dance Videos

English Country Dancing Documentary: Accessed March 8, 2015,
    https://www.youtube.com/watch?v=YO7SBhCg_AQ
Emperor of the Moon. English Country Dance: Accessed March 8, 2015,
    https://www.youtube.com/watch?v=IKnV4wQ3Sr0
May Pole Dance: Accessed June 3, 2013,
    http://www.youtube.com/watch?v=BtT21X4gKsM&feature=fvwrel

Music and Dance Trivia

Who were the Beatles?
An English rock band formed in Liverpool in 1960.

Who are the Rolling Stones?
An English rock band formed in London in 1962. The first settled line-up consisted of Brian Jones, Ian Stewart, Mick Jagger, Keith Richards, Bill Wyman, and Charlie Watts.

Who is Phil Collins?
An English singer, songwriter, multi-instrumentalist, and actor who became famous as both the drummer and lead singer for the rock group *Genesis*, plus he gained worldwide fame as a solo artist.

Who is Dizzee Rascal?
An English hip-hop musician.

Who is Richard Thompson?
Music critics consider him one of the best acoustic guitar players of all time. Thompson was also one of the first to blend English folk music and electric guitar styles.

Who is Boy George?
A singer-songwriter who was part of the English New Romantic movement which emerged in the late 1970s to the early 1980s.

Who was David Bowie?
An English singer, songwriter, multi-instrumentalist, record producer, arranger, and actor.

Who is Elton John?
Sir Elton Hercules John is an English singer, songwriter, composer, pianist, record producer, and occasional actor.

Who is Bernie Taupin?
An English lyrist who has been Elton John's songwriting partner since 1967. They have collaborated on more than 30 albums.

Who is Sophie Ellis-Bextor?
An English songwriter and singer who rose to prominence as the lead singer of *Theaudience* in the late 1990s. She went solo after the group disbanded and became a prominent UK female singer in the early 2000s.

Food

British food has traditionally been based on beef, lamb, pork, chicken, and fish and is generally served with potatoes and one vegetable. The most common foods eaten in Britain include the sandwich, fish and chips, pies such as the cornish pasty, trifle, and roast dinners.

The staple foods of Britain are meat, fish, potatoes, flour, butter, and eggs. Many American dishes are also based on these foods. Native food grown in England includes wheat, barley, corn, rye, oats, rapeseed, sugar beets, alfalfa, and clover as well as apples, pears, plums, black currants, cauliflower, and cabbage. Sheep are raised in the countryside and oyster farming and fresh water fishing are popular.

Recipe

Yorkshire Pudding. This is a traditional food served at a family Sunday brunch. Yorkshire pudding is served with the meal, filled with gravy and vegetables. Any pudding left over at the end of the meal is served cold with jam or ice cream as a dessert. It is never re-heated. Serves six.

Ingredients.
4 large eggs
Milk and flour each equal to the volume of the eggs
Pinch of salt

2 tablespoons of lard, beef dripping, or vegetable oil.

Preparation. Heat the oven to 450 degrees F. Pour eggs, flour, salt, and milk into a bowl and mix with an electric mixer. Let stand 10 minutes. Then make sure all the lumps are removed and let stand for a minimum of 30 minutes (you can let this sit several hours).

Place a drop of lard into a 4" by 5" baking pan and heat the pan in the oven until the lard smokes. Re-mix the batter after adding two tablespoons of cold water. Put the lard, drippings, or oil in the pan. Fill the pan with the batter and return it to the oven. Cook for about 20 minutes, until the pudding is golden brown. Serve hot with gravy and vegetables.

Food Trivia

What is Yorkshire pudding?
A main dish made from flour, eggs, and milk, baked, and served with gravy.

What is a traditional way to eat a Yorkshire pudding?
Fill each pudding with gravy and vegetables for dinner. After dinner, any unused puddings can be served with jam or ice cream as a dessert.

What is toad-in-the-hole?
Sausages covered in batter and roasted.

What are fish and chips?
Flour-battered deep-fried cod, haddock, huss, or plaice. Served with deep-fried potatoes similar to French Fries. Topped with malt vinegar.

True or false: Fish and chips are usually cooked at home.
False: Fish and chips are England's traditional take-out food.

What is a chippie?
A fish-and-chips shop.

What is a ploughman's lunch?
A piece of cheese, a bit of pickle and pickled onion, and a chunk of bread.

What is cottage pie?
A dish made with minced beef and vegetables and topped with mashed potato.

What is bubble and squeak?

A meal made from leftover vegetables and meat. Usually cabbage, peas, carrots, and Brussels sprouts are fried in a pan with mashed potatoes and meat until brown. The name comes from the sounds the food makes as it is being cooked.

What is the original main ingredient in pie and mash?

Jellied eels. Until about 50 years ago they were cheaper than beef. Today most are made with beef.

Customs

Weddings

If the bride sees the groom before she gets to the church on her wedding day, it's bad luck.

A bride must not wear her veil or both shoes to the church. These must be put on only after she arrives and is ready to walk down the aisle. If she does this, she gets good luck.

A bride kissed by a chimney sweep on her way to the church will have good luck.

After the wedding, the groom carries the bride over the threshold to avoid evil spirits gathered at the doorway.

Traditionally the bride and groom drank mead, a drink made of fermented honey, for a month after the wedding to assure a successful marriage.

A lunar month is a full cycle of the moon. Each full moon has a name with the honey moon occurring most often in June. The honeymoon was the traditional time after the wedding for celebration.

Children

It was traditional to drink *posset*, hot milk mixed with alcohol and spices, out of specially spouted *posset* kettles to encourage a pregnant woman's body to start labor. The idea was that the milk would replenish the mother's flagging energy and the alcohol would numb her pain. This is no longer done.

Holidays

January 1: New Year's Day.
Variable date: Good Friday
Variable date: Easter.
Day after Easter: Easter Monday.
May 1: May Day.
Last Monday in August: Summer Bank Holiday.
December 25: Christmas.
December 26: Boxing Day.
December 31: New Year's Day.

Customs Trivia

True or false: Seeing a black cat is good luck.
True.

True or false: White heather is lucky.
True.

What should you say for good luck on the first day of the month?
White rabbit, white rabbit, white rabbit.

What do you do in the autumn for good luck?
Catch falling leaves.

What do you do to make a wish come true?
Touch wood.

What do you do if you spill salt?
Toss some over your shoulder to avoid bad luck.

What happens if you pass someone on the stairs?
Bad luck.

Why do you put a spoon in the bottom of an empty egg shell?
To chase the devil away.

What is the reason bread doesn't rise?
There is a dead body nearby.

Why cut off the ends of the bread before serving?
To make the devil fly away from the house.

More Resources

DVDs

Discovering England, DVD, Questar, 2001.
Passport to England, Ireland and Scotland, DVD, Travel Channel, 2004.
Rick Steve's England and Wales, DVD, Perseus, 2009.
Ultimate England, DVD, Pilot Productions, 2006.

Books

Campbell, K. *United Kingdom in Pictures* (Lerner Publications, 2004).
Else, D. *England Country Travel Guide* (Lonely Planet, 2011).

Websites

Welcome to gov.uk: Accessed December 29, 2015. www.direct.gov.uk/
Visit England: Accessed December 29, 2015, www.enjoyengland.com/

Photos

England Photos: Accessed April 5, 2015,
    http://www.picturesofengland.com/
England Pictures: Accessed April 5, 2015, http://www.earth-
    photography.com/Countries/England
England. Pictures: Accessed April 5, 2015,
    http://www.tripadvisor.com/LocationPhotos-g186217-England.html
Exploring the most picturesque & historic parts of England: Accessed
    April 5, 2015, http://www.picturesofengland.com/
Historic England: Accessed April 5, 2015,
    http://www.imagesofengland.org.uk/

References

Dating and Marriage Customs in England: Accessed June 29, 2012,
    http://www.woodlands-junior.kent.sch.uk/customs/questions/dating.htm
English Americans: Accessed December 29, 2015,
    http://en.m.wikipedia.org/wiki/English_American

England: Accessed March 8, 2015,
  http://www.travelmath.com/from/Seattle,+WA/to/London,+United+Kingdom

England Forever. Music: Accessed March 8, 2015,
  http://www.englandforever.org/england-music.php

English Country Dancing: Accessed March 8, 2015, http://www-
  ssrl.slac.stanford.edu/~winston/ecd/origins_and_evolution.htmlx

Famous English Americans or Celebrities of English Descent: Accessed March 8, 2015,
  http://www.imdb.com/list/ls051382680/

Famous People from England: Accessed December 29, 2015,
  http://barryruterford.hubpages.com/hub/Famous-People-from-England

Famous Landmarks Found in England: Accessed December 29, 2015,
  http://projectbritain.com/landmarks.htm

Geography and Map of the United Kingdom: Accessed December 29, 2015,
  http://geography.about.com/library/cia/blcuk.htm

Greensleeves: Accessed December 29, 2015,
  http://www.songfacts.com/detail.php?id=8685

Greensleeves lyrics: Accessed December 29, 2015,
  http://www.smartlyrics.com/Song291069-Folk-Songs-Greensleeves-lyrics.aspx

Interesting Facts about England: Accessed March 8, 2015,
  http://www.eupedia.com/england/trivia.shtml

London Hotels: Accessed March 8, 2015, http://www.tripadvisor.com/Hotels-g186338-
  London_England-Hotels.html

May Day: Accessed December 29, 2015, http://projectbritain.com/mayday.htm

Music of Yesterday: Accessed March 8, 2015, http://musicofyesterday.com/history/new-
  history-english-music/

Narrative History of England: Accessed March 8, 2015,
  http://www.britannia.com/history/narprehist.html

Some Crazy British Sports: Accessed March 8, 2015,
  http://www.funtrivia.com/en/subtopics/Some-Crazy-British-Sports-272399.html

Ten Most Popular Sports in England: Accessed March 8, 2015,
  http://sporteology.com/top-ten-popular-sports-uk/

Top Ten Most Famous English Singers: Accessed March 8, 2015,
  http://www.toptenfamous.com/top-10-most-famous-british-female-singers/

Typical Traditional English Dishes: Accessed March 8, 2015,
  http://resources.woodlands-junior.kent.sch.uk/customs/questions/food/dishes.htm

FINLAND

Basics

Geography

Finland is bordered by Sweden, Russia, the Baltic Sea, the Gulf of Bothnia, and the Gulf of Finland. The country's size is 130,127 square miles, slightly smaller than the state of Montana. It is a mostly flat land, more than 70 percent covered by thick forest. In the southern areas there are countless clearwater lakes.

Language

The principal languages spoken in Finland are Swedish and Finnish. Immigrant languages include Arabic, Chinese, English, Northern Kurdish, Polish, Romanian, Russian, Somali, Tatar, Turkish, and Vietnamese.

History

The history of Finland began in about 7000 BC with Stone Age humans and by 2500 BC farming communities were established. There is little or no evidence that Finns ever had contact with Greece or Rome.

In the Middle Ages, Christian missionaries arrived and converted the people. During this time, the Danes invaded Finland twice and the people who are today's Russians attempted to conquer the land.

Swedish colonists migrated to Finland in such large numbers that in 1323 AD Finland became a province of Sweden. The Union of Norway, Sweden, and Finland dissolved in 1523 AD.

During the winter of 1696-97 a severe famine reduced the population of Finland by about a third. This was followed by the Great Northern War of 1709-21 when Russians invaded and occupied the country. In 1710 a plague reached Helsinki and devastated the population.

In 1809 the Finns accepted Tsar Alexander of Russia as their ruler. Finland would become a Grand Duchy rather than a part of Russia.

In the late nineteenth century Finnish nationalism began to grow and in 1858 the first Finnish-speaking grammar school opened. In 1902 Finnish was made an official language along with Swedish.

Finland became an independent Republic in 1917. In April 1918 German troops captured Helsinki but were eventually defeated and in 1919 Finland again gained independence.

Finland became involved in the Second World War when Russia invaded in 1939. In 1940 Finland was forced to surrender the southeast area including the city of Viipuri and territory north of Lake Lagoda. In 1942 Finland joined with Germany in attacking Russia and recaptured their territory, but after the war Finland was forced to surrender large amounts of territory to Russia.

After the collapse of the Soviet Union in 1991, the treaty of 1947 was replaced by a new treaty in 1992 in which both sides agreed to settle their differences in a friendly manner.

Map and Flag

Flag of Finland. Accessed June 27, 2015,
   http://www.enchantedlearning.com/europe/finland/flag
Map of Finland: Accessed June 27, 2015,
   http://www.worldatlas.com/webimage/countrys/europe/lgcolor/ficolo
   rlf.htm

Travel

Distance

From New York, NY, to Helsinki is 4,123 miles. Flight time is 8 hours 45 minutes.

From Chicago, IL, to Helsinki is 4,440 miles. Flight time is 9 hours 23 minutes.

From Dallas, TX, to Helsinki is 5,231 miles. Flight time is 10 hours 58 minutes.

From Seattle, WA, to Helsinki is 4,718 miles. Flight time is 10 hours 4 minutes.

Hotels

Fabian Hotel. Located in Helsinki. Wheelchair-accessible, allows dogs, its staff are multilingual, and it has wonderful views of the city.

GLO Hotel Art. Located in Helsinki near art museums. It has in-room mini-bars and provides laundry service.

Hotel Haven. Located in Helsinki, it has 77 luxury rooms, a gym, free breakfast, and conference rooms available.

Hotel Kamp. Located in Helsinki, it has a golf course and a spa, and offers smoking and non-smoking rooms.

Scandic Paasi. Located in Helsinki its rooms have kitchenettes, there is an on-site restaurant, and it offers children's activities.

Landmarks

Fortress of Suomenlinna. Located at the entrance to Helsinki's harbor, it has protected the country since the eighteenth century.

Helsinki Cathedral. Located in Helsinki, it was built as a tribute to Russian Tsar Grand Duke Nicholas I and, before the independence of Finland in 1917, it was known as St. Nicholas' Church.

Koli National Park. Located in eastern Finland, it features natural boreal forests, silicate-rock vegetation, herb-rich forests, highland and lowland meadows, eskers, and bog woodlands.

Lapland. The home of Santa Claus Village, an amusement park located in the northern part of the country near the town of Rovaniemi on the Arctic Circle. The site offers views of tundra and pine forests.

Rauma. A UNESCO World Heritage Site best known for its high-quality lace and the Old Town for its old wooden architecture. The fifth largest port in Finland.

Travel Trivia

What is the official name of Finland?
The Republic of Finland.

True or false: Finland is the most sparsely populated country in the European Union.
True.

What is the capital of Finland?
Helsinki.

What is the highest point in Finland?
Halti Mountain at 4,344 feet.

How many lakes does Finland have?
Over 188,000.

Why is Finland called the Land of the Midnight Sun?
During the summer the sun does not drop below the horizon.

True or false: There are no pay phones in Finland.
True. Finland is the home of Nokia, the largest cell-phone manufacturer in the world.

What cell phone game was created in Finland?
Angry Birds.

How much does a traffic ticket cost in Finland?
It depends on how much you earn.

What form of relaxation is common in Finnish homes?
A sauna.

What do most people in Finland do immediately after a sauna?
Jump into a lake.

Where can visitors stay during Finnish winters?
A rented igloo.

What must drivers do during daylight hours?
Headlights must be on all day long.

What is the Päijänne Water Tunnel?
Europe's longest tunnel and the world's second longest.

True or false: There are no one-cent coins in Finland.
True. Amounts are rounded to the closest five cents.

At what age do children start school?
Age seven. And they do not receive grades in school until eighth grade.

Who is Saint Henry of Finland?
The patron saint of Finland, an English bishop who arrived with Swedish crusaders in the twelfth century.

When did prohibition come to Finland?
Kieltolaki (prohibition) was in force from 1919 to 1932.

What was the original form of money in Finland?
In the fifth century Finns bought and sold goods using squirrel skins.

What weapon was invented in Finland?
The Molotov cocktail, during World War II.

America's Roots

Who is Marissa Mayer?
The CEO of Yahoo. Her mother is from Finland.

Who was Eero Saarinen?
Born in Finland, he came to the United States at age 16 and became a famous architect. He designed the Gateway Arch in St. Louis.

Who is Jean M. Auel?
The author of *Clan of the Cave Bear*. Both of her parents were born in Finland and she was born in Chicago.

Who is Matt Damon?
The American actor's maternal grandparents are from Finland.

Who is Jessica Lange?
The American actress' mother was born in Finland.

Who is Christine Lahti?
The American actress' paternal grandparents immigrated to the United States from Finland.

Who is Jorma Kaukonen?
A member of the rock band *Jefferson Airplane* whose paternal grandparents were from Finland.

Who is Vampira?
An actress who was born in Finland and came to the United States at age 2 years. She starred in the movie *Plan 9 From Outer Space*.

Who was Buffalo Bill Cody?
A Western showman, his paternal grandfather came from Finland.

Who is Timothy L. Kopra?
An American astronaut with Finnish ancestors.

Who is Linus Torvalds?
The Finnish creator of the Linux computer operating system.

Who was Jean Sibelius?
A world-famous Finnish composer.

Who is Renny Harlin?
A Hollywood director of Finnish descent.

Who is Tapio Wirkkala?
A Finnish glass designer.

Who is Esa-Pekka Salonen?
A world famous conductor.

Sports and Games

Sports

The national sport of Finland is *pesäpallo*, meaning *nest ball* and sometimes called Finnish baseball. It is a combination of traditional ball-batting team games and North American baseball.

The game is played when one team tries to score by hitting the ball and running through the bases, and the other team tries to defend by catching the ball and putting the runners out. The most important difference between *pesäpallo* and baseball is that the ball is pitched vertically. This makes hitting the ball, as well as controlling the power and direction of the hit, much easier. Other popular sports include floorball, Nordic walking, running, and skiing.

Floorball is a form of floor hockey. It is played with five players and a goalkeeper on each team. Men and women play indoors using a perforated plastic ball and a hockey stick. A match is 23 minutes long.

Nordic walking, created in 1979, is fitness walking using specially designed walking poles. Walkers apply force to the poles with each stride and use more of their entire body than in normal walking.

The country is home to many skiers and has produced Olympic-winning skiers in cross country and downhill skiing.

The Finnish enjoy watching motor sports such as rally driving and participating in folk racing. Folk racing competitions are divided into classes depending on age and gender, and participants can be as young as 15. The race is divided into heats, usually with six cars. To keep the sport available to the average person, all the cars have the same nominal value and, after a race, any competition-licensed driver can make a bid on any car. If there is more than one offer for a car, the buyer is chosen randomly. Refusing to sell your car is grounds for having your competition license revoked.

Ice hockey is the most popular sport in Finland, both as a professional and an amateur sport. There are about 68,000 registered players, 430 clubs, 3,000 teams, and 40,000 amateur games played each year.

Sports Trivia

True or false: Wife-carrying is a Finnish sport.
True. And you can compete with a woman who is not your wife. The winner gives the carried woman her weight in beer.

Who was Lauri "Tahko" Pihkala?
He invented pesäpallo in the 1920s.

What is the only sport Finland has won at the Summer Olympics since 1900?
The javelin throw. Finland has enjoyed success in this sport from the 1900s to the present day.

Who was Veli Saarinen?
Winner of one Olympic gold and three World Championship titles in the 1920s and 1930s in cross-country skiing.

Who was Veikko Hakulinen?
Winner of three Olympic gold medals and three World Championship gold medals in the 1950s and 1960s in cross country skiing, as well as a World Championship silver medalist in biathlon.

Who was Juha Mieto?
He won an Olympic gold medal in 1976 and two overall FIS Cross-Country Skiing World Cups.

Who is Marjo Matikainen-Kallström?
She won a gold at the 1988 Winter Olympics, three World Championships, and three overall World Cups in cross country skiing.

Who is Marja-Liisa Kirvesniemi?
She won three gold medals at both the Olympics and World Championships and two overall World Cup titles in cross country skiing.

Who is Kalle Palander?
She was Slalom World Champion in 1999 and World Cup Slalom champion in 2003 as well as the Alpine Skiing World Cup.

Who is Tanja Poutiainen?
She won three World Cup titles in Slalom and Giant Slalom in the 2000s.

Game

Crab Ball Tag. A traditional game in Finland, here modified for residents

Number of players. Eight.

Materials. A large ball and a table around which are seated the residents.

To play. Residents push the ball with their heads towards one another. The player who hits the ball off the table is out.

Winner. The player who remains at the end of the game is the winner.

ICHI benefits. Physical joint movement, voluntary body movement, control of body movement, and mental functions of language.

Music and Dance

Music

The history of music in Finland begins with *runolaulu*, a form of epic poetry with vocal harmony. The poems of the *Kalevala*, first published in the nineteenth century, combined folklore and mythology, and gave Finnish music a distinct sound.

Stringed instruments such as the *kantele* and the *jouhikko* are unique to Finland.

The creation of the Kaustinen Folk Music Festival in 1968 helped to revive interest in Finnish folk music. In 1983, the band Värttinä formed and began *a cappella* performance of traditional folk songs and the Kalevala.

Modern Finland's music scene features folk musician troupes who are pushing the boundaries of the genre. Exploring the possibilities of fusing the soulful sounds and epic stories of folk with other styles, many musicians are combining folk music with other national music as well as genres such as rock, gypsy, jazz, and even tango.

Music Videos

Finnish Folk Music: Accessed June 27, 2015,
    https://www.youtube.com/watch?v=j1a4bNn1FEs
Finnish woman playing the *kantele*: Accessed June 27, 2015,
    https://www.youtube.com/watch?v=dYFh_WjWrYk
The Finnish *Kantele*: Accessed June 27, 2015,
    https://www.youtube.com/watch?v=9cRXOhqOFEM
Three Finnish Folk Instruments: Accessed June 27, 2015,
    https://www.youtube.com/watch?v=HuuDQOyUqDU
Värttinä: Accessed June 27, 2015,
    http://www.worldmusic.net/guide/finland-new-runes

Dance

Pelimanni is folkdance music which usually features the accordion and fiddle. It is found throughout all of the Nordic countries but has particular prominence in Finland.

The oldest known traditional dances in Finland are *caroles*, simple chain dances in which a linked line of dancers moves forwards, walking, running, or skipping while singing. The dances are simple and depend on the leader of the chain, who leads the dancers along a labyrinthine path over the floor, curving round, twisting, and turning back, sometimes going under arched arms. Other formations are also used: simple circles, squares, and lines are popular; featuring movement around the circle or going forwards and backwards in the line and changing places. Although the dancers are not divided into couples, in some ring dances one couple might perform in the middle for a while. The dance and the song are not connected with each other and any song could be used for any figure. The leader usually starts a narrative ballad and the dancers join in with him. There is traditionally no instrumental accompaniment. Chain dances have been in Finland for a long time, especially at weddings, where they have been used as ritual dances up to the present century.

Purpuri are long ceremonial dances, containing elements of many different types of dance and usually starting and ending with a march. As wedding dances, this style could last for hours.

Finnish folk dances differ from those in other European countries in several ways. There are no men-only or women-only dances and both sexes have always enjoyed dancing together. There are also no sword-dances or show-dances where men perform for attention.

Dance Videos

Finland Folk Dance. Lappi Lapland: Accessed June 27, 2015,
    https://www.youtube.com/watch?v=TCBsvg-LbLw
Finnish Ballet: Accessed June 27, 2015,
    https://www.youtube.com/watch?v=s-gM67EK8Vs
Finnish Folk Dances: Accessed June 27, 2015,
    https://www.youtube.com/watch?v=j3rDbejHJ_g
Tango from Finland. Eurovision Dance Contest 2008: Accessed June 27, 2015, https://www.youtube.com/watch?v=k76hu07zqJE
The Snow Queen. Finnish Ballet: Accessed June 27, 2015,
    https://www.youtube.com/watch?v=cPueD4uIjx4

Music and Dance Trivia

What is the Sibelius Academy?
Located in Helsinki, it is considered one of the best music universities in Europe.

Who is Karoliina Kantelinen?
A member of Värttinä and a teacher at Sibelius Academy.

What is a *kantele*?
A traditional plucked string instrument in the dulcimer and zither family.

What is a *jouhikko*?
A traditional, two- or three-stringed, bowed lyre with strings traditionally made of horsehair.

What is a *pitkähuilu*?
A long flute used in Finland for about 2,000 years.

What is a *puusarvi*?
A wood horn traditionally played by women.

What is a *säkkipilli*?
A bagpipe used in Finland during the middle ages.

What is a *pikkuliru*?
A clarinet-like instrument used by herders in Karelia.

What is Piirpauke?
A band whose music combined jazz with traditional Finnish music.

What is Kardemimmit?
A famous quartet of female Finnish singers who perform folk songs.

What is the Finnish tango?
A version of the Argentine tango adapted by the Finnish in the 1930s.

How is the Finnish tango different from the Argentine tango?
It uses a beguine rhythm during the chorus and a habanera rhythm.

What instruments are used for the Finnish tango?
Accordion and drums.

Who is Jorma Elo?
He is a contemporary choreographer born in Helsinki in 1961.

What is the Finnish National Ballet?
A professional ballet company in Helsinki, founded in 1922.

Who is Sorella Englund?
A former soloist and character dancer with the Royal Danish Ballet.

Who was August Bournonville?
A Danish ballet master and choreographer who worked with many Finnish dancers.

Who is Tero Saarinen?
A Finnish dance artist, choreographer, and the artistic director of *Tero Saarinen Company*.

Who was Alina Frasa?
Born in Finland in 1834, she is regarded as the first ballerina in Finland.

Who is Anu Viheriäranta?
A Finnish ballet dancer who joined the Dutch National Ballet in 2005 and became a principal dancer in 2010.

Food

Traditionally Finnish people eat food originating straight from the fields, lakes, and forests, including fish, meat, mushrooms, and grains such as rye, barley, and oats. They also eat berries, including strawberries, blueberries, lingonberries, and cloudberries. Milk and potatoes are popular as well as root vegetables and cabbage.

Finnish breakfast usually consists of open-faced sandwiches. The sandwich is often buttered and topped with hard cheese or cold cuts. The lunch menu is often soup made of peas and fish. Dinner may also include soups as well as meats and larger fish portions.

Recipe

Finnish Squeaky Cheese. A favorite breakfast item in Finland.

Ingredients.
2½ gallons milk
1 tablespoon salt

1 tablespoon cornstarch
1 tablespoon sugar
½ rennet tablet

Preparation. Heat milk in double boiler to 88 degrees F. (be careful not to exceed 90 degrees). Dissolve crushed rennet in 1 tablespoon of cool water and set aside. In a cup, mix dry ingredients with a small amount of the warmed milk. Add this mixture and the dissolved rennet to the rest of the warmed milk. Stir well and set aside to gel. Do not disturb. Gelling time varies from 20 to 45 minutes. Test by inserting wooden spoon gently into mixture. When jelled properly, the spoon should leave a clean hole.

When gelled, stir to break up curds into 1" chunks. Let set for 5-10 minutes, until whey separates from curds. Set out a 9" round cake pan with a thin, wet cloth draped over it. Pour jelled mixture onto cloth, then gather all corners and squeeze out as much whey as possible. Remove cloth carefully and firmly press the mass into pan.

Bake at 400 degrees F. for 15 minutes, periodically pouring whey off. Broil on both sides until light golden-brown. Cool on rack and let dry for 1-2 hours. Refrigerate.

Food Trivia

What is a favorite Finnish beverage?
Milk.

Why do Finns eat rye bread?
It was a food created by the poor but now is eaten as a health food.

What is meat stew?
A traditional meat-and-potato stew.

What are popular stew meats?
Pork, beef, and reindeer.

How are potatoes traditionally served?
Boiled or mashed.

What is lingonberry marmalade?
A topping served on potatoes.

Why do the Finnish eat so much fish?
They live in a land of over 188,000 lakes and enjoy creamy fish soups.

Who eats porridge?

Everyone of every age. Porridge is eaten topped with berries and grains.

What is a favorite Finnish dessert?

Oven-baked cheese with cloudberry sauce.

What is a traditional Finland Christmas dinner?

Ham with mustard, potatoes, vegetable casserole, beetroot salad, carrots, apples, sweet Christmas bread, homemade cheese, and pies filled with rice and meat and served with broth.

Customs

Weddings

Traditional marriage in Finland began with a discreet inquiry to see if a marriage proposal would be accepted. A Finnish suitor was then accompanied by a spokesman who presented the man and his case for marriage. When the bride-to-be made her appearance, a bottle of spirits and other gifts were given. Receiving gifts didn't mean a binding acceptance because the gifts could be returned if the groom was rejected. If the answer was favorable, the girl and her parents visited the suitor's parents' home. The future daughter-in-law might also stay for a week and help with the household work.

The majority of Finns to this day still belong to the Lutheran Church. Church weddings remained compulsory until approximately 1917. Today, couples marry in a church or civil venue, and sometimes even in shopping centers. The bride traditionally wears a white wedding dress and veil or headdress. The groom wears a dark suit.

It is Finnish tradition for the bride to walk down the aisle alongside the groom and then stand together in front of the celebrant. However, many twenty-first century brides choose to be given away by the bride's father or an older male relative.

At the reception, a boy may be placed on the bride's lap for a short while to encourage fertility. Dancing with the bride is a tradition. The last dance of night is a traditional waltz, which starts off with all of the women dancing in turn with the bride, while the men dance with the groom. At some point, a swap is made, with the idea that before the end of the dance, every man, woman, and child will have danced with the bride and the groom.

It is also traditional for both bride and groom to sit on special seats of honor at the reception. As guests pay their respects, they would deposit cash gifts into a shawl-covered sieve held by the bride. The Finnish alternative to throwing the bouquet to identify the next potential bride-to-be is the passing-on of the bridal crown. The single women blindfold the bride and then dance around her. The bride has to grab one and successfully pass over her bridal crown, as a fun way to find the next bride!

Wedding festivities include musical chairs. Children's party games may also be part of the fun, with special celebratory prizes such as champagne.

Children

When a baby is born in Finland, the newborn is greeted with small gifts from friends and family which are either brought at the first visit in hospital or home or sent to the home. It is customary to bring or send flowers to the mother and a small token, such as a soft toy, to the child.

In Finland every newborn receives a box of gifts from the state, a starter kit of clothes, sheets, and toys in a box that can even be used as a bed. Mothers have a choice of taking the starter kit or a cash grant of about US$190. Ninety-five percent of new mothers choose the box which is worth much more.

Originally created for low-income families, the starter kit became available to all parents in 1949. Since then, it's been a staple of new parenthood and a sign that no matter what their background, all Finnish babies will get an equal start in life.

On the child's first birthday, family and relatives are invited to the family home for coffee. Parties including other children begin at age 3 or 4 years. For young children, the party is usually at home. For older children, the party can be at home or in some other location, such as an adventure park, on a ship, in a museum, or in a restaurant.

Holidays

January 1: New Year's Day.

January 6: Epiphany.
Variable date: Good Friday.
Variable date: Easter.
The Monday after Easter: Easter Monday.
May 1: May Day.
Variable date: Ascension Day.
Variable date: Whit Sunday.
June 20: Midsummer holiday.
October 31: All Saints' Day.
December 6: Independence Day.
December 25: Christmas.
December 26: St. Stephen's Day.
December 31: New Year's Day.

Customs Trivia

What is the bride-stealing game?
A tradition in which the bride is whisked away by the groomsmen and held ransom until the groom completes a special task in order to get her back.

Why do the bride and groom stomp the floor?
Whoever stomps first asserts their status as the boss of the household.

What do guests traditionally do at the wedding reception?
Make speeches.

What type of wedding cake is served?
The wedding cake includes fresh cream, fruit, and berries.

What is the wedding-cake custom?
The bride and groom feed each other a piece of cake to symbolize their willingness to nurture each other.

How long are Finnish couples usually engaged?
Three to four years.

How long is the woman called a bride?
It was customary for a newlywed bride to be known as the bride until her first child was born. Only then does she become a wife.

Who does the bride give a gift to on the second day of her marriage?
Her mother-in-law.

More Resources

DVDs

7 Days Finland, DVD Travel Video Store. Amazon Instant Video, 2007.
Global Treasures Olavinlinna St. Olaf's Castle Finland, DVD.
    TravelVideoStore. Amazon Instant Video, 2009.
Global Treasures Porvoo Finland, DVD. TravelVideoStore. Amazon
    Instant Video, 2009.
Nature Wonders Lemmenjoki Finland, DVD. Travel Video Store.
    Amazon Instant Video, 2007.
Vista Point Helsinki Finland, DVD. TravelVideoStore. Amazon Instant
    Video, 2007.

Books

Ross, Z. *Finland* (Insight Guides, 2014).
Saxon, L. *Guide to Finland and Scotland: A World of Learning at Your
    Fingertips* (Smart Kids, 2015).
Steves, R. *Rick Steves' Snapshot St. Petersburg, Helsinki, & Tallinn* Rick
    Steves, 2013).
Symington, A. *Finland TravelGuide* (Lonely Planet, 2015).

Websites

Finland: Accessed June 27, 2015,
    http://www.state.gov/r/pa/ei/bgn/3238.htm
President of the Republic of Finland: Accessed June 27, 2015,
    http://www.presidentti.fi/public/default.aspx?nodeid=44845&content
    lan=2&culture=en-US
Republic of Finland: Accessed June 27, 2015,
    http://www.nationsonline.org/oneworld/finland.htm
The Official Travel Site of Finland: Accessed June 27, 2015,
    http://www.visitfinland.com/

This is Finland: Accessed June 27, 2015,
http://finland.fi/Public/default.aspx?

Photos

Finland: Accessed June 27, 2015,
http://www.lonelyplanet.com/finland/images
Finland: Accessed June 27, 2015,
http://travel.nationalgeographic.com/travel/countries/finland-guide
Finland Pictures: Accessed June 27, 2015,
http://www.tripadvisor.com/LocationPhotos-g189896-Finland.html
Finland. Pictures of the Best Country: Accessed June 27, 2015,
https://www.youtube.com/watch?v=u4V6eTCE3YA
Finland's Ten Most Beautiful Landscapes: Accessed June 27, 2015,
http://www.visitfinland.com/article/finlands-ten-most-beautiful-landscapes

References

12 Fascinating Traditions for Welcoming Newborns: Accessed June 27, 2015,
http://www.oddee.com/item_98850.aspx
A Short History of Finland: Accessed June 14, 2015,
http://www.localhistories.org/finland.html
Finland: Accessed June 14, 2015,
http://www.nationsencyclopedia.com/economies/Europe/Finland.html
Finland Culture for Children: Accessed June 27, 2015,
http://dinolingo.com/blog/2012/06/07/finland-culture-for-children-childrens-games-of-finland/#.VY7ZcflViko
Finland Hotels: Accessed June 22, 2015, http://www.tripadvisor.com/SmartDeals-g189896-Finland-Hotel-Deals.html
Finland Squeaky Cheese: Accessed June 27, 2015,
http://www.foodgeeks.com/recipes/finnish-squeaky-cheese-leipajuusto-3808
Finland's Best Folk Festivals: Accessed June 27, 2015,
http://theculturetrip.com/europe/finland/articles/the-finnish-folk-renaissance-finland-s-best-folk-festivals
Finland Travel Math: Accessed June 22, 2015,
http://www.travelmath.com/from/Dallas,+TX/to/Helsinki,+Finland
Finnish Sports in Finland: Accessed June 27, 2015, http://www.expat-finland.com/events/finnish_sports.html
Finnish Wedding Traditions: Accessed June 27, 2015,
http://www.worldweddingtraditions.net/finnish-wedding-traditions

Fun Facts About Finland Travel 2008-2015: Accessed June 27, 2015,
    mhttp://www.venere.com/blog/15-fun-facts-about-finland
Interesting Facts About Finland: Accessed June 27, 2015,
    http://www.eupedia.com/finland/trivia.shtml
Languages of the World: Accessed June 14, 2015,
    http://www.ethnologue.com/country/FI
Nine Famous Finnish Americans. Accessed June 27, 2015, http://cassavafilms.com/list-
    of-9/nine-famous-finnish-americans
Old Marriage Customs in Finland: Accessed June 27, 2015,
    http://sydaby.eget.net/swe/jp_marriage.htm
Purpurit Finnish Folk Dance: Accessed June 27, 2015,
    http://vcn.bc.ca/purpurit/finnish_folk_dance.htm
Sport in Finland: Accessed June 27, 2015, https://en.wikipedia.org/wiki/Sport_in_Finland
Ten Amazing Facts About Finland: Accessed June 27, 2015,
    http://www.finnbay.com/media/homebred/10-amazing-facts-about-finland
Ten Strange Historical Facts About Finland: Accessed June 27, 2015,
    http://www.historyextra.com/feature/animals/10-strange-historical-facts-about-
    finland
The Music of Finland: New Runes: Accessed June 27, 2015,
    http://www.worldmusic.net/guide/finland-new-runes
Traditional Finnish Food: Accessed June 27, 2015,
    http://www.slideshare.net/kaukajarvi/traditional-finnish-food-17687018
Traditional Finnish Musical Instruments: Accessed June 27, 2015,
    http://www.forumbiodiversity.com/showthread.php/28038-Traditional-Finnish-
    Music-Instruments
Wally Huskonen, "Some Famous Finnish-Americans," *Collecting Ancestors* (blog),.
    August 21, 2014, http://www.collectingancestors.com/2014/08/21/some-famous-
    finnish-americans
Why Finnish Babies Sleep in Cardboard Boxes: Accessed June 27, 2015,
    http://www.bbc.com/news/magazine-22751415
World Tourist Attractions 2012: Accessed June 27, 2015,
    http://thetouristattractions.blogspot.com/2012/07/5-best-tourist-attractions-in-
    finland.html

FRANCE

Basics

Geography *how many have visited France*

France is about 80 percent of the size of Texas, but its landscape is not anything like Texas. It is the home of Europe's highest mountain, Mont Blanc, at 15,781 feet and of the Vosges Mountains which are covered in forests. The country has four river basins and a plateau. Three flow west, the Seine into the English Channel, the Loire into the Atlantic, and the Garonne into the Bay of Biscay. The Rhine flows south into the Mediterranean.

Language *how many can speak some French*

French is spoken in France, and in more than 25 countries formerly governed by France. The earliest evidence of the language comes from the Strasbourg Oaths of 842 AD. The Paris dialect, *Francien*, has been the official standard language since the mid-sixteenth century.

History

Cave art tells researchers that pre-modern hominid populations lived in France between 30,000 and 10,000 years ago. Greek and Phoenician traders traveled along the French Mediterranean coast after about 600 BC and Celts migrated westward and settled in the area.

Julius Caesar conquered the area, then called Gaul, in about 52 BC and it remained Roman until the fifth century AD when the Franks invaded. In the eighth century AD, King Charlemagne consolidated territory and called himself the Holy Roman Emperor. After his death, his three grandsons divided his territory into what eventually became France, Germany, and Italy.

In 1328 France, under King Philip VI, was the most powerful nation in Europe with a population of 15 million. Twenty years later the Black Death, bubonic plague, killed approximately one-third of the country's inhabitants.

The country's fortunes reversed as they rebuilt. King Louis XIV built the Palace of Versailles as a celebration of French art and architecture. However, his overspending and the economic troubles of the country's poor led to the French Revolution which lasted from 1789 to 1794.

The ideals of the revolution seemed short-lived with the rise of Napoléon Bonaparte who reigned from 1804 to 1814. He was followed by Louis-Philippe from 1830 to 1848 and then the Second Empire of Napoléon III from 1852 to 1870. The Franco-Prussian War ended the rule of Napoléon III and ushered in the Third Republic which lasted until France's military defeat at the hands of Nazi Germany in 1940.

France suffered huge losses in World War I. The horror was repeated in 1940 when Nazi Germany invaded Paris. The country was liberated by the Allies in 1944. The nation then began losing its grip on its foreign territories. Morocco and Tunisia received independence in 1956, French West Africa in 1960, and Algeria in 1962.

Map and Flag

Flag of France: Accessed March 27, 2015,
   http://www.coloringcastle.com/flag_coloring_pages.htm
Map of France: Accessed March 27, 2015,
   http://www.coloring.ws/france.htm

Travel

Distance

From New York, NY, to Paris is 3,363 miles. Flight time is 7 hours 46 minutes.

From Chicago, IL, to Paris is 4,143 miles. Flight time is 8 hours 47 minutes.

From Dallas, TX, to Paris is 4,940 miles. Flight time is 10 hours 23 minutes.

From Seattle, WA, to Paris is 5,010 miles. Flight time is 10 hours 31 minutes.

Hotels *has anyone stayed in one of these*

Hotel Regina. Located at 2 Place Des Pyramides in Paris, within walking distance of the Museum of Decorative Arts, the Louvre Museum, and the Palais Royal. It features premium linen-dressed beds.

Hotel Renaissance Paris Arc de Triomphe. Located at 39 Avenue de Wagram in Paris, just a short walk from the Arc de Triomphe, Champs-Elysees, and the Musée d'Art Moderne de la Ville de Paris. Its beds are dressed in premium cotton sheets.

Les Jardins du Marais. Located at 74 Rue Amelot in Paris, it is a nineteenth century building near the Picasso Museum.

L'Hotel du Collectionneur Arc de Triomphe. Located at 51-57 Rue de Courcelle in Paris, it overlooks the Parc de Monceau and has a health club where hotel guests can work with a personal trainer and enjoy a hydrotonic bath, a massage, and beauty treatments.

Normandy Hotel. Located at 7 Rue De L'echelle in Paris, its rooms are furnished with antiques and breakfast is served daily.

Landmarks

Arc de Triomphe. Located in Paris near the Eiffel Tower, it was built to honor those who fought and died for France during the French Revolution and the Napoleonic Wars. Work began in 1808, commissioned by Napoleon, and was completed 28 years later. Underneath the Arc de Triomphe is the Tomb of the Forgotten Soldier where an eternal flame commemorates those fallen in World War I.

Cité de Carcassonne. Located in the southern Languedoc-Roussillon region of France, this medieval fortification has 52 towers. For over 2,500 years the walls have withstood the changes of politics and war and in 1997 it was named a UNESCO World Heritage Site.

Dune of Pyla. Europe's tallest sand dune. Located on France's west coast, it is estimated to contain 60,000,000,000,000,000 grains of sand — enough sand to fill 338,142,471,000 teacups.

Eiffel Tower. Constructed in 1889 as a gateway to the Exposition Universelle, a World's Fair. It was scheduled to be torn down in 1909, but the French government decided to use it to send out radio signals and it remains a symbol of France. The tallest building in Paris, visitors can climb its hundreds of steps or ride in an elevator for an amazing view of the city.

Louvre. This museum is housed in the *Palais du Louvre*, the former seat of French royalty. Beginning as a twelfth century fortress, it became a public art museum during the French Revolution. It has become the world's most-visited museum with eight thematic departments and 35,000 works of art dating from antiquity to the early modern period, including works by European masters such as DaVinci, Delacroix, Vermeer, and Rubens, as well as unsurpassed Greco-Roman, Egyptian, and Islamic arts collections. *what's a favorite painting?*

Mont Blanc. Located in the Alps, half in France and half in Italy, it is the largest peak in Europe. Climbers scale it with and without guides while others ride cable cars for a view of the mountain.

Notre Dame Cathedral. Located in Paris, this has been called the most stunning Gothic cathedral in the world. Work on the cathedral started in the twelfth century and was completed two centuries later. It was the center of medieval Paris and became famous worldwide when novelist Victor Hugo set *The Hunchback of Notre Dame* there. Visitors can climb the north tower for a one-of-a-kind view of Paris.

Travel Trivia

Who was France's first female prime minister?
Edith Cresson, who served from 1991 to 1992.

What is *Chambord*?
A grand home which some historians believe may have been partially designed by Leonardo Da Vinci. Its construction started in 1519 and it was never fully completed. King François I used it as a hunting lodge in the sixteenth Century.

What is the Sorbonne?
One of Europe's oldest universities, it was founded by Robert de Sorbon, Louis IX's chaplain, and opened in 1253 to provide quarters for theology students who were not friars.

What is the Palace of the Popes?
Located in Avignon, construction began in 1305 when Pope Clement V, who was French, decided to establish his papal court in France. Construction continued until 1377 when Pope Gregory XI brought the Avignon papacy to an end and returned the papal court to Rome.

True or False: France is the third largest country in Europe.
True. It is third in size after Russia and Ukraine.
what 2 countries are larger

What is Europe's oldest canal?
The Canal du Midi, which was built between 1666 and 1681, is 150 miles long, and includes 63 locks, 126 bridges, 55 aqueducts, 7 canal bridges, 6 barrages (small dams), and one tunnel.

Where are the strongest tides in Europe?
Between Brittany and Normandy where the difference between high and low tide can be 15 meters (49 feet).

What is the highest town in Europe?
Briancon, France, which is located at an altitude of 3,175 meters (10,400 feet).

Where is the largest canyon in Europe?
Verdon Gorge in France is the largest in Europe and second largest in the world, at 25 kilometers long and 700 meters deep.

What was the world's first common international language?
French, which was spoken in Europe, across the Ottoman Empire, and was the official language of England from 1066 to the fifteenth century. In the mid-twentieth century French was replaced by English as the most common international language.

How many French citizens speak more than one language?
A 2005 study found that 45 percent speak a second language, with 34 percent choosing English as their second language.

Is the French spoken in Quebec, Canada, the same as in France?
No. Quebec has a distinct dialect which is hard for French speakers to understand.

True or false: France is the last European country to use checks.
True. Checks were phased out in other European counties in the 1990s as they were considered security risks.

What are some famous inventions credited to France?
The adding machine, the hot air balloon, the airship, the parachute, the submarine, ambulance services, and photography.

Which country holds the largest number of Nobel Prizes for Literature?
France, with 13 as of January 2015.

Where and when was the world's first scientific conference held?
Paris, France, on February 2, 1799.

Where can you find hundreds of crocodiles relaxing in France?
The Crocodile Farm in Pierrelatte, because of the hot water provided by the nearby Tricastin Nuclear Power Center.

What is France's chief energy source?
France was the first producer of nuclear electricity in Europe and second producer in the world after the United States. France produces as much nuclear electricity as Germany, the United Kingdom, Spain, and Russia combined.

True or false: France has the third highest per capita hourly income in the world.
True. US$38.16 per hour. Norway and Luxemburg are first and second, respectively.

True or false: The French were the first to produce commercial wine and liquor.
True.

America's Roots

Who was Henry Wadsworth Longfellow?
A poet of French descent who wrote *Paul Revere's Ride*, *The Song of Hiawatha*, and *Evangeline*. His first major poetry collections were *Voices*

of the Night in 1839 and *Ballads and Other Poems* in 1841. Longfellow died in 1882.

Who was John Greenleaf Whittier?

A writer and abolitionist who became a newspaper editor during the 1830s. In 1833 he published the antislavery pamphlet *Justice and Expediency*. He was a founding member of the American Anti-Slavery Society and when he spoke out against slavery he was often stoned. His ancestors were French Huguenots.

Who was Henry David Thoreau?

Born in 1817, he is famous for *Walden*, a diary of his life while spending two years in a wilderness near Concord, Massachusetts. His ancestors were French.

Who was Edna St. Vincent Millay?

A poet and playwright, she received the 1923 Pulitzer Prize for Poetry for *The Harper Weaver and Other Poems*. Her talent first became apparent when, at age 14, she won the St. Nicholas Gold Badge for poetry. Her ancestors were French.

Who was Robert Goulet?

An actor who made his debut in the Broadway production of *Camelot* in 1960. At age 14 he won a singing scholarship to the Royal Conservatory of Music in Toronto. He earned a Tony award in 1968 for *Happy Time* and performed for three US presidents and Queen Elizabeth II. His parents were French-Canadian.

Who was Maurice Jarée?

A composer who won several Academy Awards in the 1960s for his musical scores for such classic American films as *Lawrence of Arabia*, *Dr. Zhivago*, *Grand Prix*, and *The Longest Day*. He was a French American.

Who was Ron Turcotte?

A jockey who rode the most famous American racehorse of all time, Secretariat, to victory in the Triple Crown of horse racing. His ancestors were French.

Who was Thomas Gallaudet?

In 1817 he founded the first American school for the deaf in Hartford, Connecticut. He also founded teacher-training schools and believed in and promoted advanced education for women. After his death in 1851, Gallaudet College, a national institute for the deaf, was established in Washington, DC, in 1855. He was born in Pennsylvania of French descent.

Who was James Bowdoin?

A governor of Massachusetts and first president of the American Academy of Arts and Letters. He also founded Bowdoin College and established the Massachusetts Humane Society. He grandfather was a French Huguenot.

Who was John Jay?

A politician born in New York City in 1745, the writer of *The Federalist Papers,* and the first US Chief Justice. He served as president of the Continental Congress and negotiated the treaty with England that ensured American independence. He was of French descent.

Who was Paul Revere?

A gold- and silversmith who joined the Freemasons and launched the Boston Tea Party revolt. He later was made famous in the poetry of Henry Wadsworth Longfellow for riding to Lexington on April 18, 1775, at 10 pm to warn John Hancock and Samuel Adams of the approaching British army. He was of French descent.

Who was Matthew Fontaine Maury?

The father of modern hydrography, he was born in 1806 near Fredericksburg, Virginia. From 1825 to 1834 he made first three voyages around the world, to Europe, and to the Pacific coast of South America. His ancestors were French Huguenots.

Who is Warren Edward Buffett?

A businessman and philanthropist, he is the chairman and largest shareholder of Berkshire Hathaway and in 2008 was listed as the wealthiest person in the world. He has pledged to give 99 percent of his wealth to charity. He has French ancestors.

Who was Franklin Parsons "Frank" Perdue?

He was president and CEO of Perdue Farms, one of the largest chicken-producing companies in the United States. In over 200 commercials, he branded himself by saying, "It takes a tough man to make a tender chicken." He had French ancestors.

Who is René Murat Auberjonois?

An actor known for playing roles such as Father Mulcahy in the film version of *M*A*S*H*, Clayton Endicott III in *Benson*, and Odo in *Star Trek: Deep Space Nine*. He has French ancestors.

Sports and Games

Sports

One of the best known international sporting events, the Tour de France, takes place in France. It is a cycling competition that takes place every July and lasts three grueling weeks. It requires cyclists to master rough terrain over 2,235 miles, even in rain, which can be quite treacherous.

The most popular sport in France, as in most of Europe, is football, which Americans call soccer. France won the World Cup in 2006. There are amateur football clubs in every town, including clubs for children as young as age 3 years. This sport usually attracts males while young girls play volleyball, hockey, and basketball.

Second in popularity is tennis, and the country hosts world competitions at Roland Garros. The last Frenchman to win the French Open was Yannick Noah in 1983.

Handball became popular in the early 1990s. The French team won the bronze medal at the 1993 Summer Olympics, reached the finals of the 1993 World Championship, and finished third in the 2005 Summer Olympics. Handball is also popular in primary and secondary schools in France.

France has won the rugby Six Nations Championship 14 times, played against England, Ireland, Italy, Scotland, and Wales.

An American sport growing in popularity in France is basketball. The national basketball team falls under the jurisdiction of the Fédération Française de Basket-Ball.

Card games are popular in France. There are local games but when it comes to international games, bridge is the favorite with over 80,000 members in the national federation. The French are also fans of poker and rummy, plus a unique French style of Poker called *Courchevel*.

Sports Trivia

Who is Mary Pierce?
Winner of the 2000 French Open.

Who is Jeannie Longo-Ciprelli?
A cyclist who won a gold medal in the 1966 Summer Olympic Games and a silver medal in the 1962 Olympic Games. She won French and World Championship cycling titles 51 times.

Who is Thierry Henry?
A soccer player who became a professional at age 17. In 2004 and 2005 he won the European Golden Boot award. He is also the top scorer for Arsenal, both in the Premier League as well as in European cups including the Champions League.

What is grand randonnees?
The term for long distance walking trails in France.

What is the rule when walking trails in France?
It is an offense to leave the trail to walk on the grass.

What is *boules* or *petanque*?
Lawn bowling. Two teams attempt to roll or throw balls closest to a jack in the middle of the field, knocking their opponent's ball out of the way. In Italy the game is call *bocce*.

Why did the Tour de France begin?
Over 100 years ago a journalist created and sponsored the race simply to increase circulation for his newspaper.

What is *parkour*?
A form of running in which obstacles in the landscape are not avoided but quickly navigated by jumping, leaping, quick crawling, and climbing.

Who created *parkour*?
A French teenager in the late 1980s.

What is a French mountain-climbing challenge?
Climbing to the summit of Mont Blanc in the French Alps. This may take 10-12 hours.

Game

Bilboquet has been popular in France since the sixteenth century.

Number of players. One per cup. This can be used as a solitary game for one resident or with up to six residents in competition.

Materials. For each player: string, a large bead with a hole through the center, scissors, and a paper cup.

To play. String the string through the bead and punch a hole at the bottom of the cup with the scissors. Next, pull the string through the hole and tie a knot so the string is attached to the cup. Using only one hand, players try to swing the bead into the cup.

Winner. The first one to get their bead into the cup.

ICHI benefits. Control of voluntary movements, muscle force, and mobility of joints.

Music and Dance

Music

The history of French music begins in the tenth century with court songs and chivalrous music. Much of France's early folk music was instrumental, using very few and very simple instruments.

Modern French music history begins in the early 1600s with the introduction of French opera and French classical music. In the beginning, most of the music was holy songs from the Roman Catholic Church. But soon French musicians began to write about love. The nineteenth century was the beginning of the French romantic era in both songs and film.

The most famous romantic French singer is Edith Piaf, whose 1945 ballad *La vie en rose* won a Grammy Hall of Fame Award in 1998. She became famous as an entertainer in France even before the Second World War, then worked internationally and performed at Carnegie Hall.

While the purity of French music lies in its classical and folk tunes, more recent chapters in the history of French music include pop and hip-hop-style beats.

Folk music in France is regional with no single timeline. In the south, the folk music resembled Spanish or Italian folk music, and in the eastern mountains, Swiss or German influences played a role in folk music. The north of France and the Atlantic Coast each had fairly individualized genres of folk music that were part of local community and artistic life.

France is the only country in Europe where national music is two-thirds of all music sold and the law has a part in this trend. Radio stations must play a minimum of 40 percent French music as stipulated by a law passed in 1986. The amount required can range from 25 to 60 percent depending on a station's particular broadcasting policy.

Music Videos

Best Classic French Songs: Accessed March 11, 2015,
    https://www.youtube.com/watch?v=5mAtVsA-pes
Best French Music for a Romantic Dinner: Accessed March 11, 2015,
    https://www.youtube.com/watch?v=5mAtVsA-pes
French Music in the French Café: Accessed March 11, 2015,
    https://www.youtube.com/watch?v=s6BuZOYboZM

Dance

France has been the cultural center of Europe since medieval times and the French style of ballet was born during the time of Louis XIV. (Ballet itself began in fifteenth century Italy.) Dancing was a popular pastime for the king and ballroom and square dances were also popular, not just in royal circles but also in community halls where local residents joined in dance.

The *gavotte* was a popular dance in a two-step and a hop pattern, commonly performed to the music of Bach. The rigaudon is another lively Baroque dance found in music halls until the nineteenth century. After Louis XIV opened the first-ever ballet school in 1661, it became possible to train professionally in France.

The *can-can* arrived in Paris about 1830 as a couples' dance including a series of high kicks. There was a movement to ban the dance and men doing a *can-can* would be arrested, but the dance continued to grow in popularity. *Can-can* chorus lines arose in the United Kingdom and the United States, and were later imported to France for the benefit of tourists.

Folk dances are regional with Celtic influences apparent in the use of bagpipes and hurdy-gurdys as musical instruments.

Dance Videos

French Can-Can Dance: Accessed March 30, 2016,
  www.youtube.com/watch?v=OddjQA4q1_M
French Folk Dance: Accessed March 11, 2015,
  https://www.youtube.com/watch?v=cQdwg_cbfuk
How Great is Our God. Paradosi Ballet Company: Accessed March 11,
  2015, https://www.youtube.com/watch?v=cQdwg_cbfuk5

Music and Dance Trivia

What French song recorded by Frank Sinatra is popular in the United States?
Autumn Leaves, known in Frances as *Les Feuilles Mortes*, written by Yves Montand.

> *The falling leaves drift by the window*
> *The autumn leaves of red and gold*
> *I see your lips, the summer kisses*
> *The sunburned hands I used to hold*
>
> *Since you went away the days grow long*
> *And soon I'll hear old winter's song*
> *But I miss you most of all my darling*
> *When autumn leaves start to fall*

Who was Claude-Achille Debussy?
A famous composer born in 1862 who learned to play the piano at age 7 and four years later was admitted to the Paris Conservatoire. His most famous works are *The Afternoon of a Faun* and *Children's Corner*.

Who was Victor Hugo?
Born in 1802, he wrote *Les Miserables*. In 1851 Hugo was exiled for speaking out against Napoleon III. He returned to France in 1870 and was greeted as a national hero.

Who was Jean-Jacques Rousseau?
A philosopher and composer born in 1712. His writings form the basis of socialism, liberal thought, and nationalism, and influenced the French Revolution. He was also a composer and a music theorist.

Who was Claude Monet?
One of the pioneers of Impressionist painting, he was born in 1840. The term *Impressionism* was derived from the name of one of his paintings, *Impression, Sunrise*. One of his most famous paintings is *Water Lilies* which he created in a garden he designed.

Who is Brigitte Bardot?
One of the world's most famous actresses. Born in Paris in 1934, she began modeling in her early teens and appeared in her first movie in 1952. Throughout the 1950s and 1960s she was considered a sex symbol and made bikini swimwear popular. In the 1970s she retired from films to become an animal-rights activist.

Who was Charles Pierre Baudelaire?
A French poet born in 1821 who became fascinated with Edgar Allen Poe. In 1857 he wrote *The Flowers of Evil*, a series of poems about death, ugliness, and beauty. His work was not appreciated until after his death in 1867.

Who was Jules Verne?
He was born in 1828 and became the father of science fiction. He wrote 54 novels including *20,000 Leagues Under the Sea*, *A Journey to the Center of the Earth*, and *Around the World in Eighty Days*, all futuristic scenarios based in scientific fact. He is the second-most translated author in the world.

Who was Adolphe Adam?
A composer who wrote the ballet *Giselle*, first performed in Paris in 1884. The ballet is the story of the spirit of a woman who died before her wedding day of a broken heart yet returned as a ghost to save her former love.

Food

Seventeen percent of France is used for agriculture and the country is the leading crop exporter in the European Union. The foods grown and exported by France includes apples, cherries, pears, grapes, pumpkins, olives, asparagus, cabbage, artichokes, sugar beets, mushrooms, wheat, barley, and corn.

The French love preparing, serving, and enjoying good food. There are some dishes the French are known for around the world, including *coq au vin*, a chicken fricassee cooked in red wine with mushrooms and sometimes garlic, and *crêpes* which are flat pancakes typically stuffed with fruit or cream. There is also the *baguette* which is a long French bread loaf.

French desserts are a real treat. Some well-known desserts are *mousse* which is a light chocolate pudding that originated in France, the *éclair* which is a pastry stuffed with cream and topped with icing, and *crème brûlé* which is a custard topped with broiled caramel.

Most French people eat bread, wine, and cheese daily. In fact, on average each person in France eats 45 pounds of cheese per year. There are about 400 kinds of French cheese, all classified by the type of milk (goat, cow, or ewe), whether or not the milk was pasteurized, and how the cheese was pressed.

Recipe

Baguette. This bread is a staple of the French diet, often served with cheese or with a meal.

Ingredients.
1 package dry yeast
1 tablespoon salt
2 tablespoons sugar
2½ cups warm water
7 cups flour
1 egg white, lightly beaten

Preparation. Grease two cookie sheets. In a large mixing bowl, dissolve the yeast, salt, and sugar in the warm water. Stir in the flour until a stiff dough forms. Turn the dough onto a floured surface and knead for 10 minutes.

Clean out the mixing bowl, lightly oil it, and return the dough to the bowl. Cover the bowl with plastic wrap. Let the dough rise until doubled in size, about 30 minutes or so. Dip your fist in flour and push your fist into the center of the dough to punch it down. Remove dough from the bowl and knead 3 or 4 times. Separate the dough into 4 equal pieces. Form each piece into a long loaf. Place 2 loaves on each greased cookie sheet. Carefully slash the top diagonally every few inches with a sharp knife. Brush the loaves with the egg white. Cover lightly with plastic wrap and let the loaves rise again for about 30 minutes. Preheat oven to 400 degrees F. Bake loaves for 10 minutes then lower heat to 350 degrees F. and bake for 20 more minutes.

Food Trivia

How long is a lunch period in France?
Lunch time is usually two hours. In large cities businesses close from noon to 2 pm when restaurants serve lunch.

How many restaurants are there in Paris?
Over 5,000.

What is the French paradox?
Scientists are puzzled by the low rate of chronic heart disease in France despite the French people having a diet high in saturated fat. Some believe that drinking red wine protects against heart disease.

If you are what you eat, what is the state of French health?
The French style of eating mostly dairy has resulted in the longest life expectancy (81.1 years) of any European Union country and a very low rate of obesity.

True or false: The French invented foie gras.
False: This dish began 4,500 years ago in ancient Egypt.

What is a truffle?
An edible underground fungus believed to be an aphrodisiac. This food is cultivated by men called *trufficulteurs*, who use trained pigs or dogs to hunt by smell for the truffles.

What was the first French cookbook?
Le Cuisine François was written by the famous French chef La Varenne in 1652.

How many new cookbooks does France produce?
On average, two per day.

Who brought the French cooking style to America?
Chef Julia Child, via her cookbook *Mastering the Art of French Cooking.*

What is nouvelle cuisine?
Developed in the 1970s, as a reaction against the classical French school of cooking. Nouvelle cuisine is simpler, portions are smaller, and cooking is quicker.

Customs

Weddings

French wedding traditions will be familiar to many in the United States, such as the wedding armoire, known as the traditional hope chest in America. It is used to store the bride's trousseau, including linen, jewelry, and clothing. It is usually made by the father of a future bride and is given to her while she is still young. Wedding armoires are usually hand-carved with symbols of wealth and prosperity. A woman is expected to fill her armoire over the years, so it will be ready to take to her new home once she marries.

One tradition still active in French villages is the wedding procession. It begins when the groom arrives at the bride's house on the morning of the wedding. He will escort her to the chapel in a procession headed by musicians, then the bride, the bride's father, family, guests, and the groom and his mother walking at the back of the line. Sometimes the bride and groom will be met by village children who tie white ribbons across the road which the bride must cut as a symbol of the couple overcoming obstacles in their marriage.

At the wedding ceremony, tradition has the bride and groom sit on two velvet chairs underneath a silk canopy known as a *carre* when they make their vows. A square of silk fabric or a veil is held over the heads of the couple during the priest's final blessing to protect the couple from evil spirits. The same silk or veil is saved and used to protect their newborn child when baptized.

The traditional French wedding cake is a *croquembouche*, invented in the seventeenth century. It is made of small, cream-filled pastry puffs which are piled in a pyramid and covered with a caramel glaze.

Children

Traditionally a child was given the name of the saint whose day coincided with the birthday of the child. Thus, parents didn't choose a name and used the name assigned to that day by the church. This is no longer done. However, many French parents will use the saint's name as a middle name.

In France, as in Greece, many people celebrate two birthdays. The first, the anniversary of the day of their birth, is celebrated with a birthday party with friends. The second, the feast day of their saint's name, is celebrated with a small, quiet dinner with family.

Birthday cake in France is a fruit tart or a chocolate mousse-filled tart, decorated with whole nuts or a French cake or tart topped with glazed fruit and cream. There is no frosting and names are not written on the dessert.

There are no baby showers for pregnant women in France. The French believed that people should wait for the baby's first birthday to celebrate the event by giving gifts to mother and baby.

Birth rituals no longer practiced in France include hanging prayer sheets or blessed medals over the cradle and drawing a chalk line around the child's house to protect the newborn child from evil.

Holidays

January 1: New Year's Day
Variable date: Good Friday
Sunday after Good Friday: Easter
Monday after Easter: Easter Monday
Day after Pentecost: Whit Monday
May 1: May Day
May 8: Victory in Europe Day
July 14: Bastille Day
November 11: Armistice Day
December 25: Christmas

December 26: St. Stephen's Day
December 31: New Year's Day

Customs Trivia

What must a wife avoid to prevent her husband from experiencing kidney pain?
A wife should never iron her husband's underpants while wearing a belt.

How can you be assured of giving birth to a girl?
A pregnant woman who sees an owl will give birth to a girl.

Why should a couple never have 13 people at a dinner?
It is bad luck because it is the number of attendees at *The Last Supper*.

Why should a bride avoid a tortoiseshell cat?
Seeing one means you will die in an accident.

How do you bring good luck into a new house?
Bring the dining table in first.

What should you wear on New Year's Day to ensure a year of good luck?
Polka-dotted clothing.

What should you do when you meet a French sailor?
Rub his beret for good luck.

Why do you never give knives as a wedding gift?
A knife as a gift means you are cutting the receiver out of your life.

What happens if you light a candle from another candle?
All you wish for will be transferred to the first person who lit the candle.

Why do the French hang good-luck horseshoes with the opening facing down?
So good luck will pour down on you.

Resources

DVDs

Globe Trekker France, DVD, 2003.
Rick Steves' Best of Travels in Europe: France, DVD, 2001.
Rick Steves' Europe: France and Benelux, DVD, 2007.
T & T's Real Travels in France, DVD, 2008.
Visions of France, DVD, 2006.

Books

Neal, L., *France: An Illustrated History* (Hippocrene, 2001).
Jenkins, C., *Brief History of France* (Running Press, 2011).
Robb, G., *Parisians: An Adventure History of Paris* (Norton, 2011).
Robb, G., *The Discovery of France: A Historical Geography* (Norton, 2008).
Horne, A., *Seven Ages of Paris* (Vintage, 2004).

Websites

France: Accessed January 4, 2015, http://www.france.fr/en.html
French food: Accessed January 4, 2015, http://www.french-culture-for-visitors.com/history-of-french-cuisine.html
French history and culture: Accessed January 4, 2015, http://www.french-property.com/reference/french-history
French Tourism: Accessed January 4, 2015, http://francetourism.com
Discover France: Accessed January 4, 2015, http://www.discoverfrance.net/France/DF_govt.shtml

Photos

Free digital photos of France: Accessed January 4, 2015, http://www.freedigitalphotos.net/images/France_g144.html
Free downloadable photos of Paris: Accessed January 4, 2015, http://www.world-city-photos.org/Paris
Free photos of Paris: Accessed January 4, 2015, http://www.world-city-photos.org/Paris/photos/Eiffel_Tower

Free printable photos of France: Accessed January 4, 2015,
    http://www.world-city-photos.org/Paris
Photos of Paris: Accessed April 2, 2015,
    http://photobucket.com/images/paris%20france

References

Alpine Ibex: Accessed January 3, 2015, http://www.lhnet.org/alpine-ibex
Autumn Leaves lyrics: Accessed January 3, 2015, http://www.metrolyrics.com/autumn-
    leaves-lyrics-frank-sinatra.html
Card Games in France: Accessed January 3, 2015,
    http://www.pagat.com/national/france.html
Edna St. Vincent Millay: Accessed January 3, 2015,
    http://www.everyculture.com/knowledge/Edna_St__Vincent_Millay.html
Eurotunnel: Accessed January 2, 2015,
    http://www.eurotunnel.com/uk/inspiration/ideas/Top-Landmarks-in-France
Famous French People: Accessed January 3, 2015,
    http://www.buzzle.com/articles/famous-french-people.html
Food in Every Country: Accessed January 3, 2015,
    http://www.foodbycountry.com/Algeria-to-France/France.html
France: Coloring Castle: Accessed March 9, 2015,
    http://www.coloringcastle.com/flag_coloring_pages.html
France Coloring Pages: Accessed March 9, 2015, http://www.coloring.ws/france.htm
France: Geography, History, Politics, and More: Accessed January 2, 2015,
    http://www.infoplease.com/country/france.html#ixzz3NfMcKznN
French Americans: Accessed January 3, 2015, http://www.everyculture.com/multi/Du-
    Ha/French-Americans.html
French Food Facts: Accessed March 11, 2015,
    http://www.frenchdesire.com.au/facts/food
French History: Accessed January 2, 2015,
    http://www.nationsonline.org/oneworld/History/France-history.htm
French wedding traditions: Accessed January 3, 2015,
    http://www.weddinglegend.com/french-wedding-traditions
History of French Dance: Accessed January 3, 2015,
    http://www.ehow.com/about_6584501_history-french-dance.html
History of French Music: Accessed January 3, 2015,
    http://french.lovetoknow.com/History_of_French_Music
History of French Music: Accessed January 3, 2015, http://www.visit-and-travel-
    france.com/history-of-french-music.html
How French Traditions Work: Accessed March 10, 2015,
    http://people.howstuffworks.com/culture-traditions/national-traditions/french-
    tradition7.htm
Interesting Facts about France: Accessed January 3, 2015,
    http://www.eupedia.com/france/trivia.shtml

John Greenleaf Whittier: Accessed January 3, 2015,
http://www.everyculture.com/knowledge/John_Greenleaf_Whittier.html
Notre Dame Cathedral: Accessed January 3, 2015,
http://goparis.about.com/od/sightsattractions/p/Notre_Dame.htm
Paris Hotels: Accessed March 9, 2015, http://www.expedia.com/Hotel-
Search?#&destination=Paris%20%28and%20vicinity%29,%20France&startDate=03
/10/2015&endDate=03/11/2015&adults=2
Paul Revere: Accessed January 3, 2015, http://www.biography.com/people/paul-revere-
9456172#!
Pets in France: Accessed January 3, 2015,
https://www.justlanded.com/english/France/Articles/Moving/Pets-in-France
Popular French Sports: Accessed March 10, 2015,
http://french.lovetoknow.com/Popular_French_Sports
Relations with France: Accessed January 3, 2015,
http://www.state.gov/r/pa/ei/bgn/3842.htm
Robert Goulet: Accessed January 3, 2015, http://www.imdb.com/name/nm0332587
Some Facts about French Songs: Accessed January 3, 2015,
http://www.understandfrance.org/France/FrenchSongs.html
Sorbonne: Accessed January 3, 2015, http://www.encyclopedia.com/topic/Sorbonne.aspx
The Latin Quarter: Accessed January 3, 2015,
http://goparis.about.com/od/picturesofparis/ig/Latin-Quarter-Gallery/Sorbonne-
University-.htm
The Louvre Museum in Paris Complete Information for Visitors. Accessed January 3,
2015, http://goparis.about.com/od/parismuseums/a/Louvre_Museum.htm
The Palace of the Popes: Accessed January 2, 2015, http://about-
france.com/monuments/palace-avignon.htm
Thirteen French Superstitions: Accessed March 11, 2015,
http://www.frenchaffair.com.au/explore-france/thirteen-french-superstitions
Thomas Gaullaudet: Accessed January 3, 2015,
http://www.biography.com/people/thomas-gallaudet-9305354
Traditional French Children's Games: Accessed January 3, 2015,
http://www.ehow.com/list_6733374_traditional-french-children_s-games.html
Wildlife in France: Accessed January 3, 2015, http://www.lost-in-france.com/wildlife-in-
france
William the Conqueror: Accessed January 3, 2015,
http://www.biography.com/people/william-the-conqueror-9542227#synopsis

GERMANY

Basics

Geography

Germany is located in central Europe. Surrounded by Denmark, Poland, the Czech Republic, Austria, Switzerland, France, Belgium, Luxembourg, and the Netherlands, it shares borders with the second-highest number of European countries, second only to Russia. Its area is about 85 percent of the size of California.

Germany contains tall mountains, plains, and forests. It is home to the Alps, one of the largest mountain ranges in the world. Within the Alps is *Zugspitze* which has a summit that reaches 9,718 feet, the highest point of elevation in Germany. In addition to sharing borders with neighboring land areas, Germany has miles of coastlines formed by the North Sea and the Baltic Sea. Its interior contains large tracts of forests while low-lying plains lie in the northern region.

Language

The official language of Germany is German, with over 95 percent of the population speaking German. Minority languages include Sorbian, spoken by less than one percent in eastern Germany, and North and West Frisian, spoken around the Rhine estuary by about 10,000 people.

Danish is spoken by less than one percent, mainly in the area along the Danish border. Romani, an indigenous language, is spoken by less than one percent.

Immigrant languages include Turkish, which is spoken by around 1.8 percent, and Kurdish, by 0.3 percent.

History

The region became associated with the name Germany in the first century BC during the conquest of Gaul when the Romans became aware of the ethnic and linguistic distinction between the Celts and the Germans. In 800 AD Charlemagne, as Holy Roman Emperor, ruled over a territory that encompassed large parts of Europe, including present-day Germany. During the middle ages, Germany was marked by internal fighting among local rulers.

The Peace of Westphalia in 1648 resulted in a German-speaking Europe divided into hundreds of states. In the 1790s Prussia, Austria, and Russia defeated Napoleon at the Battle of Leipzig in 1813 and drove him out of German territory. In 1815, after the Congress of Vienna, German territory consisted of only about 40 states. German unification came in 1871 following the Franco-Prussian War, when Germany was transformed into an empire under Emperor Wilhelm I, King of Prussia.

During World War I Germany's goals were to enlarge Germany by adding the territory of Belgium and Poland as well as colonies in Africa. The country was defeated in 1918. The peace settlement negotiated by Britain, France, and the US in 1919, the Treaty of Versailles, imposed punitive conditions on Germany including the loss of territory, financial reparations, and a diminished military.

In 1919 the Weimar Republic was established with a constitution that provided for a parliamentary democracy in which the government was ultimately responsible to the people. This government was destroyed in 1933 by Adolf Hitler who formed the National Socialist German Workers' Party, or Nazi Party, replaced the Republic with an authoritarian government, and appointed himself chancellor. Hitler's aggression led to World War II.

Hitler was defeated in 1945 and the world learned of his crimes, known as the Holocaust. In the aftermath of World War II, the country was split into East and West Germany. East Germany was controlled by the Soviet Union who erected the Berlin Wall, guarded to prevent citizens from leaving. West Germany was a free democracy.

East Germany collapsed after the demise of the Soviet Union and in 1990 Germany was again a united country. In the twenty-first century, Germany is a successful economic power in Europe.

Map and Flag

German Flag to color: Accessed June 13, 2015,
http://www.coloringcastle.com/pdfs/flags/flag-germany-123.pdf
German Map to color: Accessed June 13, 2015,
http://www.worldatlas.com/webimage/countrys/printpage/printpage.
php?l=/webimage/countrys/europe/lgcolor/decolor.gif

Travel

Distance

From New York, NY, to Berlin is 3,978 miles. Flight time is 8 hours 27 minutes.

From Chicago, IL, to Berlin is 4,414 miles. Flight time is 9 hours 20 minutes.

From Dallas, TX, to Berlin is 5,218 miles. Flight time is 10 hours 56 minutes.

From Seattle, WA, to Berlin is 5,060 miles. Flight time is 10 hours 37 minutes.

Hotels

Circus Hotel. Located in Berlin, a tram stops at the front door and is perfect for seeing local historical sites.

Das Stue. Located in Berlin and just a 15-minute walk to the Brandenburg Gate. It has a pool, spa, and two restaurants.

Hotel OTTO. Located in Berlin, it is pet friendly, has a multilingual staff, and internet access.

Louisa's Place. Located in Berlin, it has large rooms equipped with kitchens and is near the Kurfürstendamm shopping area.

Pullman Berlin Schweizerhof. Located in Berlin, it has the largest indoor pool in the city as well as a gym and a spa.

Landmarks

Brandenburg Gate. This is the only surviving city gate of Berlin and symbolizes the reunification of East and West Berlin. Built in the eighteenth century, the Brandenburg Gate is the entry to Unter den Linden, the prominent boulevard of linden trees which once led directly to the palace of the Prussian monarchs.

Frauenkirche. The Church of Our Lady, located in Dresden, is a Lutheran church that was completely destroyed during World War II. The church was reconstructed using original plans from the 1720s and reopened in 2005. The city of Coventry, England, which was raided by the Luftwaffe, donated the golden cross for the dome of the church. Since its reopening, the Frauenkirche has been a hugely popular tourist attraction.

Heidelberg. This city is one Germany's most popular tourist destinations. During World War II, the city was almost completely spared by Allied bombings so it retains its baroque charm of narrow streets, picturesque houses, and the famous Heidelberg Castle.

Kölner Dom. Cologne Cathedral has been Cologne's most famous landmark for centuries. Construction began in 1248 and took, with interruptions, more than 600 years to complete.

Lindau. Located near the meeting point of the Austrian, German, and Swiss borders on the eastern shore of Lake Constance, this city has many medieval and half-timbered buildings.

Neuschwanstein. This castle is located on a rugged hill near Füssen in southwest Bavaria and was the inspiration for the Sleeping Beauty castles in the Disneyland parks. The castle was commissioned by King Ludwig II of Bavaria and is the most photographed building in the country.

Oktoberfest. Held in Munich, the largest Volksfest in the world with over 6 million visitors each year. It starts at the end of September and continues until the first weekend in October. An important part of Bavarian culture, the festival has been held since 1810.

Rügen Cliffs. Located in the Jasmund National Park in the northeast part of Rügen Island. Facing constant erosion, the chalk cliffs tower high above the Baltic Sea. The 387-foot Königsstuhl (king's chair) is the most majestic part of the cliffs. The undisturbed forests behind the cliffs are also part of the national park.

The Holstentor. One of the two remaining gates to the city of Lübeck. Built in 1464, it is now a museum and is regarded as a symbol of Lübeck.

The Romantic Rhine. The most famous section of the Rhine River, running between from Koblenz to Bingen. The Rhine carves its way through steep vineyard-covered hills topped with countless castles and ruins.

Travel Trivia

True or false: There are 35 dialects in the German language.
True.

What was the reason for the first Oktoberfest?
The wedding of Prince Ludwig of Bavaria.

True or false: Most of the Autobahn highway has no speed limit.
True. Sixty-five percent of the highway has no speed limit.

True or false: The first book was printed in Germany.
True.

True or false: German is the third most commonly taught language in the world.
True.

What percentage of the country is woodlands and forests?
Thirty-one percent.

True or false: Germany was the first country to adopt daylight savings time.
True. Adopted in 1916.

What year did the Berlin Wall come down?
1989.

What winter holiday tradition comes from Germany?
The Christmas tree.

What is the official name of Germany in German?
Deutschland.

What is the capitol of Germany?
Berlin.

True or false: Germany has the largest economy in Europe.
True.

What percentage of energy produced by Germany is from wind power?
Thirty-five percent.

How many zoos are in Germany?
141.

How many museums are there in Germany?
5,752 — more than in England and Italy combined.

Who built the Walhalla Temple?
Ludwig I of Bavaria, to commemorate great figures and events in Germany.

What is the Bayreuth Festspielhaus?
A theater built to host the operas of Richard Wagner.

True or false: Berlin has the largest train station in Europe.
True.

How many castles are there in Germany?
150.

What type of car are most taxis in Germany?
Mercedes-Benz.

America's Roots

Who was John Peter Altgeld?
He came to the United States from Germany at age three. As a lawyer and a Democratic governor of Illinois, he was active in prison reform.

Who was Hannah Arendt?
A Jewish German-born writer and political philosopher who held professorships at Berkeley, Princeton, and Chicago. One of her best-known works is *Origins of Totalitarianism*, published in 1951.

Who was John Jacob Astor?
Born near Heidelberg, he came to America in 1783 and became successful in the fur trade with the American Fur Company and later in New York real estate and banking.

Who was Walter Baade?
A German-American astronomer who made important discoveries at California's Mount Wilson and Palomar observatories related to star types, supernovas, galaxies, and the size of the universe. He also discovered many asteroids, including Hidalgo (1920) and Icarus (1949).

Who was John Jacob Bausch?
The co-founder of Bausch & Lomb, he was a German immigrant who borrowed money from Henry Lomb to expand his optical shop in Rochester, New York.

Who was Emile Berliner?
The German-American who invented the disk record, the gramophone, the telephone microphone, acoustic tile, and a light-weight aircraft engine.

Who was Hans Albrecht Bethe?
A German-born nuclear physicist who won a Nobel Prize in physics for his work on the energy sources of stars in 1967. He became a US citizen in 1941 and worked on the Manhattan Project in Los Alamos, New Mexico, to develop the first atomic bomb.

Who was Albert Bierstadt?
Famous for his dramatic paintings of the American West, he was born in Solingen, Germany, and came to the United States with his family in 1832. He grew up in New Bedford, Massachusetts.

Who was William Edward Boeing?
In 1916 he founded the aircraft manufacturing company Pacific Aero Products, which later bore his own surname, in Seattle in 1916.

Who was Wernher von Braun?
Born in Germany, during World War II he headed the German rocket testing facility at Peenemünde and was a member of the German team that developed the first self-guided liquid-fuel rocket, the A4 (V2). In 1945 the Americans brought him and many of his co-workers to the United States, and von Braun later worked for NASA where he was responsible for the development of the first American earth satellite (Explorer I) as well as the Saturn rockets. As head of the American space program in the 1960s, he played a big part in the success of the Apollo moon mission.

Who was George Armstrong Custer?
A fifth-generation German-American, a graduate of the US Military Academy, and a cavalry officer who fought in the American Civil War and later died at the infamous Battle of the Little Bighorn in Montana.

Who was Albert Einstein?
A German-born scientist who published his famous *Special Theory of Relativity* in 1905. He won a Nobel Prize in 1921.

Who was Dwight D. Eisenhower?
An American president whose German ancestors came to America in the 1700s. After serving as Allied supreme commander during World War II, Eisenhower became the thirty-fourth US president.

Who was Harvey S. Firestone?
The founder of the American tire and rubber company that bears his name. His German ancestors came to America in the 1700s.

Who was August Charles Fruehauf?
A German-American blacksmith who invented the tractor-trailer (semi-trailer) in 1914. Four years later he later founded the Fruehauf Trailer Corporation.

Sports and Games

Sports

The most popular sport in Germany is soccer, called *König Fußball* which means *king football*. There are thousands of amateur soccer clubs and, as a spectator sport, soccer draws an average of over 25,000 fans to each professional game.

Germany has won the soccer world championship, the World Cup, three times, in 1954, 1974, and 1990, and hosted the 2006 World Cup.

Formula One (F1) racing is very popular in Germany. A beloved sports hero is Formula One race driver Michael Schumacher, nicknamed *Schumi* by his fans, who was the top sports money earner in the world in 2004, earning about US$80,000,000 in winnings. He has earned more victories and more championships than any other F1 racer.

Tennis was very popular in Germany in the past, but interest has declined since 2000 and the sport no longer draws large crowds to events. Golf is popular with two major German European Tour golf tournaments: the BMW International Open which is held in Munich and the Mercedes-Benz Championship which is held in Pulheim near Cologne.

Ice hockey is one of Germany's most popular professional sports. It began in Berlin in 1888 and gradually spread across the country. In 1910, Germany's national ice hockey team participated in the European championships for the first time. During and after the two World Wars, Germany was banned from international hockey. The first postwar German professional ice hockey league formed in 1948. When the country was divided, there were ice hockey leagues in East and West Germany but ice hockey was not considered an important sport in East Germany.

Sports Trivia

Who is Franz Beckenbauer?
Considered the greatest German football player, he is regarded as one of the brightest stars the game has ever seen. He started his professional career in Bayern Munich in 1964 and for the next 13 years made 427 appearances and scored 60 goals.

Who is Boris Becker?
He is considered the greatest German tennis player ever. At age 17 he won the Wimbledon tournament. In his 15-year career Becker won Wimbledon three times, the Australian Open twice, and the US Open once.

Who is Katarina Witt?
She is a two-time Olympic Gold Medalist in figure skating and the champion of many European and world competitions.

Who is Wolfgang Behrent?
He is a retired amateur boxer who won a gold medal at the 1956 Summer Olympics.

Who is Oliver Kahn?

A soccer player who started his professional career in 1987, he won three World's Best Goalkeeper and four Best European Goalkeeper awards. Kahn was awarded the Golden Ball as the best player in the 2002 World Cup, the only goalkeeper ever to receive this prize.

Who was Max Baer?

A famous boxer who in 1929 fatally hurt an opponent and then decided to end his boxing career after 70 wins.

Who is Steffi Graf?

She started playing tennis at age 13 and won over 20 Grand Slam tournaments during her career.

Who is Dirk Nowitzi?

The second German player in the NBA, he plays for the Dallas Mavericks as a forward.

Who was Honus Wagner?

A German baseball player who won the World Series in 1909 and was also one of the first to be inducted in the Baseball Hall of Fame.

Who was Jurgen Klinnsman?

He started his soccer career at age 17 with the Stuttgarter Kickers. When he retired from the game, he began a second career as the manager of Germany's national team.

Game

Topfschlagen. This traditional German game is modified here for use with residents.

Number of players. Five to ten.

Materials. Plastic flower pot, candy or other treat, blindfold, and a yardstick.

To play. Residents in wheelchairs sit in a circle with a 20-foot diameter. Place the flower pot containing a treat in the center of the circle. Blindfold one resident, have an activity person roll the resident to within three feet of the flower pot, give the resident the yardstick, and let them attempt to knock over the flower pot.

Winner. The resident who successfully knocks over the flowerpot gets the treat.

ICHI benefits. Mental function of language, voluntary control of body movements, mobility of joints, and muscle force.

Music and Dance

Music

When most people think of German music, it's the classics. Germany's reputation as an important musical nation is still based on names like Bach, Beethoven, Brahms, Handel, and Richard Strauss. There are 80 publicly financed concert halls in Germany.

However, music didn't stop centuries ago. The Berlin Philharmonic, under the star British conductor Sir Simon Rattle, is considered to be the best of around 130 symphony orchestras in Germany. Frankfurt's *Ensemble Modern* annually presents over 70 new contemporary works, including 20 premieres.

The country has also experienced the 1970s disco trend, the 1980s rap and hip-hop frenzy, and the 1990s techno style. The German pioneers of electronic music, Karlheinz Stockhausen and opera composer Hans Werner Henze, have influenced contemporary music since the mid-twentieth century. The country is also home to punk rockers Die Toten Hosen and the heavy-metal band Rammstein. The teen fan group Tokio Hotel also comes under the category of German superstars.

Traditional folk music in Germany became strong under a united country in the 1800s. During the twentieth century, children in East and West Germany were taught folk songs in school, but only happy songs to inspire national pride.

Yodeling is one of the most famous stereotypes of German folk artists, but is only found in certain parts of southern Germany today. The popularity of Bavarian folk music reached its height between 1880 and the 1920s, mainly consisting of humorous songs performed in duet or ensemble.

Volksmusic and *Oompah* music are two traditional music styles. *Volksmusic*, which originated in the mountainous region of southern Germany, translates as music of the people and is played on guitars or harmonicas primarily in Bavaria. *Oompah* is played by brass bands and gets its name from the thump-thump-thumping of the tuba.

Music Videos

German Beer Song: Accessed June 13, 2015,
   https://www.youtube.com/watch?v=Y5ryo-cd-EU
German Folk Music: Accessed June 13, 2015,
   https://www.youtube.com/watch?v=8bzziAv9o4w
Good Old German Music: Accessed June 13, 2015,
   https://www.youtube.com/watch?v=q3O0aai0ACQ
Oktoberfest Music: Accessed June 13, 2015,
   https://www.youtube.com/watch?v=ii-qdSPkCfs
The Best of Classical Music: Accessed June 13, 2015,
   https://www.youtube.com/watch?v=jgpJVI3tDbY

Dance

Traditional dance is very regional in Germany. *Der Deutsche* is a traditional German dance from the mid-eighteenth century in which couples dance in circles to a tune in 3/4 or 3/8 time. *Zwiefacher* is a dance mainly known in Bavaria in which a couple dances closely together. The name can be loosely translated as twice or double time. It can be danced to over 100 different tunes.

Schuhplattler is a dance that is mainly connected to Bavaria, and often performed in traditional Bavarian costumes. During this dance, which was originally used to woo women, the men clap their hands, slap their thighs, and jump in rhythm with the music.

Maypole dances are unique to each village. The most common form of Maypole dance in Germany is the *Bandltanz*, translated as the dance of ribbons. During the dance both men and women dance around the Maypole and in the process weave together the ribbons that hang from the top of the Maypole.

Dance Videos

German Dance: Accessed June 13, 2015,
   https://www.youtube.com/watch?v=ddy4LJCC7bk
German Slap Dancing. The Fighting Dance: Accessed June 13, 2015,
   https://www.youtube.com/watch?v=2LEAiGDw220
How to Do German Dance: Accessed June 13, 2015,
   https://www.youtube.com/watch?v=DFb7nuw-5NY

Optical Illusion Dance: Accessed June 13, 2015,
https://www.youtube.com/watch?v=WeX5wuMl7lk
Pramtaler Platter: Accessed June 13, 2015,
https://www.youtube.com/watch?v=EY-ry_b5I0I

Music and Dance Trivia

What is the *Landler*?
This couples' dance was popular in the eighteenth century.

Who was Kurt Jooss?
A popular and influential German ballet dancer.

True or false: German *Schwanensee* ballets began in Germany.
False: The dance is from Russia but very popular in Germany.

What are flying steps?
A popular contemporary street dance in Germany.

Why was dance banned in Bavaria during the eighteenth century?
Dance was banned for about 30 years because authorities feared it would lead to immoral behavior.

What is the *Grossvater Tanz*, which translates as Grandfather's Dance?
A seventeenth-century German dance tune usually played at weddings.

What is the Folkwang University of the Arts?
A German institute for music, theater, dance, design, and academic studies, and home of the dance company Folkwang Tanz Studio.

What is the connection between dance and romance in Germany?
In olden days young people could only meet a future spouse at a dance.

What is traditional folk dance attire in Germany?
Dirndl dresses for the girls and knickerbockers for the boys.

What is *Zillertaler Hochzeitsmarsch*?
A Southern Germany wedding dance.

How did the Nazis use swing music?
They used modified versions of swing in Nazi propaganda to convince youths to join the Nazi party.

Who was Johann Sebastian Bach?
He is now considered to be one of the greatest German baroque composers but, while alive, he was known as an organist rather than as a composer.

What is Bach's musical heritage?
He came from a dynasty of seven generations of musicians extending from the sixteenth to the eighteenth century, with 76 male relatives who were musicians. Fifty-three of them were named Johann.

Who was Ludwig van Beethoven?
A famous classical composer who gave his first public performance at age seven and published his first work at age 12.

Who was Johannes Brahms?
A classical German composer who created four symphonies, two overtures, four concertos, piano and chamber music works, and folk song arrangements.

Who was Felix Mendelssohn?
A German composer, conductor, organist, and pianist. One of the most popular composers of the Romantic period, he was also largely responsible for inspiring interest in the music of Johann Sebastian Bach.

Who was St. Hildegard of Bingen?
An extraordinary twelfth-century Benedictine abbess who was also a composer, poet, playwright, linguist, scientist, and physician.

Who was Carl Orff?
He is best known for his cantata *Carmina Burana* and for developing the *Orff Schulwerk* (Orff Approach) of teaching music to children, a method which is used in many countries.

Who was Engelbert Humperdinck?
A nineteenth-century German composer best known for his opera *Handsel and Gretel*.

Who was Clara Schumann?
One of the top concert pianists of the nineteenth century, often considered as good as Liszt, as well as a talented composer.

Food

German food was traditionally linked to what could be grown in the short growing season of northern Europe: wheat, barley, and pasture land for livestock, supplemented by meat and/or dairy from wild game, sheep, cows, and goats. The Romans introduced the cultivation of fruit trees and grapevines. These foods remain popular today along with popular seasonings including mustard, horseradish, and juniper berries.

A menu for the average German begins with a weekend breakfast of bread, toast, and/or rolls, marmalade, honey, eggs, cold meats such as ham and salami, and various cheeses, all washed down with a strong cup or pot of tea or coffee, and usually cereals and coffee on weekdays.

Lunch is served between noon and 2 pm and is light, snack-food fare in the twentieth-first century, while dinner is usually eaten at home with the family in the evening. Traditionally, the evening meal or *Abendbrot*, meaning evening bread, consists of a selection of whole-grain bread, deli meats and sausages, cheese, and a cold or warm drink. Pork, beef, and poultry dishes as well as herring, mackerel, salmon, and sardines or freshwater fish such as trout, salmon, bream, and carp are popular. As side dishes the Germans like noodles, potatoes, and dumplings as well as red cabbage, fresh fruit, and vegetables.

Recipe

Apple Strudel. Authentic strudel is made with strudel dough, a labor-intensive, paper-thin dough. To simplify things, this recipe uses phyllo dough, which is widely available and relatively easy to work with.

Ingredients.

For the crumb mixture:

3 tablespoons unsalted butter, cut into tablespoons

1 cup fresh bread crumbs

⅓ cup sliced almonds

For the apple filling:

1½ pounds (about 4 apples) Granny Smith apples, peeled, halved, cored and very thinly sliced

1 teaspoon finely grated lemon zest

2 tablespoons lemon juice

⅓ cup golden raisins

½ cup granulated sugar
For the base:
8 sheets phyllo dough (each sheet measuring 12" x 17")
6 tablespoons unsalted butter, melted
Confectioner's sugar for sprinkling
Preparation.
Crumb mixture. In a large skillet, melt butter over medium heat. Add bread crumbs and cook over medium-high heat, stirring constantly, until crumbs are golden brown. Stir in sliced almonds and set aside to cool.

Filling. Place apples slices in large bowl and toss with lemon zest, lemon juice, and raisins. Add sugar and toss to coat.

Assemble strudel. Position a rack in center of oven and preheat oven to 375 degrees F. Lay a sheet of phyllo on a clean work surface. Lightly brush sheet with melted butter. Sprinkle with 2½ tablespoons bread crumb mixture. Layer remaining 7 sheets phyllo over first, buttering and sprinkling each one with bread crumb mixture. Spoon apple compote evenly down long side of phyllo, about 2" from bottom edge and 1" in from both sides. Fold bottom edge and side flaps over filling and roll phyllo jelly roll-style.

Transfer strudel to baking sheet and brush it lightly with melted butter. Bake for 30 to 35 minutes, or until crisp and golden. Remove strudel from oven and let cool on baking sheet placed on wire rack for 10 minutes. Dust with confectioner's sugar and slice. Serve garnished with whipped cream.

Food Trivia

True or false: Hazelnuts have been used in Germany for over 11,000 years.
True, based on archaeological pollen studies.

True or false: Beer is officially considered a food in Bavaria.
True.

How many kinds of bread are baked in Germany?
Over 300.

Where were gummy bears invented?
Germany.

How many kinds of sausage are served in Germany?
Over 1,000.

What is the proper way to order a beer in Germany?
You raise your thumb — never your index finger.

What is *marzipan*?
A sweet almond paste which can be formed into different shapes and used as a filling.

What is *stollen*?
A cake usually eaten around Christmas time, made with raisins and almonds and covered in powdered sugar.

What are *maultaschen*?
Bits of dough filled with meat, similar to ravioli and usually eaten in soup.

What is the traditional Christmas meal in Germany?
Goose.

Customs

Weddings

German law requires a civil ceremony for a marriage to be legal. Some modern couples have this small ceremony with a few friends. For those choosing a church wedding, the civil ceremony is held a few days before the church ceremony.

The engagement begins with the groom-to-be giving a gold band to the bride-to-be which she wears on her left hand and after marriage moves to her right hand. Men also wear their wedding ring on their right hand.

On the evening before the wedding friends and family gather for the *polterabend*, a party involving food, drink, and the breaking of plates and other tableware. The shattered items are cleaned up by the spouses-to-be to show that the couple will work well together. The *junggesellenabschied*, or bachelor party, is usually hosted by friends of the groom at a local pub a few weeks before the wedding.

May is the preferred month for weddings. Brides wear white gowns and grooms wear black suits. As the newly married bride and groom exit the church, rice is thrown for good luck.

A white ribbon is tied to car antennas for the procession through town. Car horns are honked during the procession. Honking back is optional. The ribbons are usually given to guests by the bride as they leave the church.

At the reception the first dance is usually a waltz reserved for the bride and groom. The second dance is for the bride and her father and the groom and his mother; the bride's mother will dance with the groom's father.

Children

Baby showers hosted by family and friends are not held for a German mother-to-be. Giving gifts to an unborn child is considered bad luck. Instead, gifts are given after the birth.

German maternity leave allows the mother eight weeks off work before giving birth and three years of unpaid time off following the birth.

Traditionally the infant was named after grandparents and great-grandparents. Each child had two names, a saint's name used during Baptism and a secular common-use name.

Holidays

January 1: New Year's Day
Variable date: Good Friday
Sunday after Good Friday: Easter
Monday after Easter: Easter Monday
First Monday in May: International Worker's Day
August 8: Peace Festival
October 3: Germany Unity Day
October 31: Reformation Day
December 25: Christmas
December 26: St. Stephen's Day
December 31: New Year's Eve

Customs Trivia

True or false: An asparagus field was often a valuable part of a German woman's dowry.
True.

What do families do when welcoming a baby girl?
They plant a tree in the front yard of the family home.

What happens to the baby girl's birth tree when she is older?
When she marries the tree is removed from the lawn and sold to help pay for her wedding.

What did a German bride traditionally carry outside on her wedding day?
Dishes. After she threw them into the street, it was considered a sign of bad luck for the marriage if a single dish remained unbroken.

What happens if a bird dies in his cage the day after the wedding?
Bad luck for the couple.

What does it mean if a bird sings on the day of the wedding?
Good luck.

What does it mean if a single person sits between the bride and groom on the wedding day?
The single person will soon be married.

What does seeing a funeral on a wedding day mean?
If the deceased is a male, the groom will die early and if the deceased is a female, the bride will die early.

Why does a pregnant woman eat apples?
To give her child rosy cheeks.

What happens if a dog frightens a pregnant woman?
The child will have a birthmark.

More Resources

DVDs

Cities of the World, Bavaria, Germany, DVD. Prime Instant Video, 2005.
Germany, DVD. Prime Instant Video, 2007.
Rick Steve's Germany and Scandinavia, DVD. Back Door Productions, 2007
Visions of Germany, DVD. Acorn Media, 2007.
Vista Point 85 Berlin Germany, DVD. Global Television, 2007.

Books

Eye Witness Travel Guide Germany (DK Publishing, 2013).
Foder's Germany. (Foder's, 2014).
Christiani, K. and A. Schulte-Peevers. *Germany* (Lonely Planet, 2013).
Christiani, K. and M. DiDuca. *Munich, Bavaria & the Black Forest*, (Lonely Plane, 2013).
Steve, R. *Rick Steve's Germany 2015* (Avalon, 2015).

Websites

German Government: Accessed June 14, 2015,
http://www.bundesregierung.de/Webs/Breg/EN/Homepage/_node.ht
ml.
German Travel: Accessed June 14, 2015,
http://www.germany.travel/en/index.html
Germany: Accessed June 14, 2015,
http://www.state.gov/r/pa/ei/bgn/3997.htm
Germany's Consulate: Accessed June 14, 2015,
http://www.germany.info/consular.
Travel information for Germany: Accessed June 14, 2015,
http://travel.state.gov/content/passports/english/country/germany.htm
l

Photos

German Photos: Accessed June 14, 2015,
 http://travel.nationalgeographic.com/travel/countries/germany-
 photos/#/germany-profile_6023_600x450.jpg
German Stock Photos and Images: Accessed June 14, 2015,
 http://www.123rf.com/stock-photo/germany.html
Germany: Accessed June 14, 2015, http://www.dreamstime.com/free-
 photos-images/germany.html
Germany's Black Forest: Accessed June 14, 2015,
 https://www.pinterest.com/deanwautier/this-is-planet-earth
Photographers of Planet Earth: Accessed June 14, 2015,
 http://photographersofplanetearth.com

References

69 Fun Facts About Germany: Accessed June 13, 2015,
 http://confessedtravelholic.com/2011/02/69-fun-facts-about-germany.html
A Guide to Folk Music Around the World: Accessed June 13, 2015, http://www.music-
 folk.com/german-folk-music/ 2011
A Short History of Germany: Accessed June 9, 2015,
 http://www.nationsonline.org/oneworld/History/Germany-history.htm
Baby Customs in Germany: Accessed June 14, 2015,
 http://www.ehow.com/info_12305288_baby-customs-germany.html
Facts About Germany. Culture and Media: Accessed June 13, 2015,
 http://www.tatsachen-ueber-deutschland.de/en/culture-and-media/main-content-
 09/cinema.html
Famous German-Americans: Accessed June 13, 2015,
 http://german.about.com/library/blfam_geramABC.htm
Famous Sports People in Germany: Accessed June 13, 2015, http://www.europe-
 cities.com/en/674/germany/sport/people
German Dance: Accessed June 13, 2015, http://www.germany101.com/page/german-
 dance
German Folk Dance: Accessed June 13, 2015,
 http://www.fitforafeast.com/dance_cultural_europe_german_folk.htm
German Food: Accessed June 14, 2015,
 http://www.braingle.com/trivia/quiz.php?id=21536
German Foods Apple Strudel: Accessed June 14, 2015,
 http://germanfoods.org/recipes/apple-strudel
Germany: Accessed June 14, 2015, http://www.howtogermany.com/pages/german-
 weddings.html
Germany Facts for Kids: Accessed June 13, 2015,
 http://www.sciencekids.co.nz/sciencefacts/countries/germany.html

History of German Dances: Accessed June 13, 2015,
http://www.ehow.com/about_6692445_history-german-folk-dance.html

Interesting Facts About Germany: Accessed June 13, 2015,
http://www.eupedia.com/germany/trivia.shtml

Introduction to German Food and Germany: Accessed June 14, 2015,
http://germanfood.about.com/od/introtogermanfood/a/introtoger.htm

Land of Ideas: Accessed June 14, 2015, http://www.research-in-
germany.org/en/discover-germany/food-and-drink/breakfast-lunch-and-dinner.html

Language, Culture, Customs and Business Etiquette: Accessed June 6, 2015,
http://www.kwintessential.co.uk/resources/global-etiquette/germany-country-
profile.html

Profiles of Great Classical Composers: Accessed June 13, 2015,
http://www.52composers.com/clara-schumann.html

Sports in Germany: Accessed June 13, 2015, http://www.german-way.com/history-and-
culture/germany/sports-in-germany

Ten Most Famous German Athletes: Accessed June 13, 2015,
http://www.mademan.com/mm/10-most-famous-german-athletes.html

The Best Hotels in Germany. Accessed June 13, 2015,
http://www.tripadvisor.com/Hotels-g187323-Berlin-Hotels.html

Top Ten Tourist Attractions in Germany: Accessed June 13, 2015,
http://www.touropia.com/tourist-attractions-in-germany

Traditional Games German Children Play: Accessed June 13, 2015,
http://www.ehow.com/list_5793665_traditional-games-german-children-play.html

Travel Math: Accessed June 13, 2015,
http://www.travelmath.com/from/Seattle,+WA/to/Berlin,+Germany

ICELAND

Basics

Geography

Iceland is located east of Greenland and immediately south of the Arctic Circle, atop the northern part of the Mid-Atlantic Ridge. It lies about 534 miles from Scotland and 2,610 miles from the United States. One of the world's most sparsely populated countries, it is the world's eighteenth-largest country in size.

Language

The official language of Iceland is Icelandic, a North Germanic language derived from Old Norse. Most residents also speak English.

History

The history of Iceland began when Celtic monks visited during the seventh and eighth centuries. The continent was settled during the ninth and tenth centuries by Norsemen from Scandinavia and Celts from the British Isles.

In 982 Erik the Red discovered and named Greenland after being banned from Iceland. Christianity came to Iceland in about 1000. Fighting between tribes then occurred until, in 1262, Icelandic chieftains accepted the sovereignty of the King of Norway. In 1387, the Kalmar Act of Union joined Iceland and Norway with Denmark.

In 1402 the Black Plague infected Iceland, resulting in over 33 percent of the population being wiped out.

In 1703 the first census was conducted: the population was 50,358. Less than ten years later, the bubonic plague wiped out one-third of the population, followed by several years of volcanic activity which destroyed Icelandic farmland and led to widespread starvation.

In 1884 the Danish king introduced a new constitution during a period of mass emigration to North America. Iceland received home rule in 1904 and in 1915 women received the right to vote.

The Union Treaty of 1918 granted Iceland full sovereignty in a royal union with Denmark. In 1926 the population reached 100,000 for the first time.

British troops occupied the country in 1940. The following year the US-Icelandic defense agreement was signed. US troops stayed in Iceland for the duration of World War II.

The Republic of Iceland was formally established in 1944 and the country joined NATO in 1949.

In 1994 Iceland joined the European Economic Area and in 2006 US troops left Iceland. In 2010 the Iceland census found there are now 296,700 people.

Map and Flag

Iceland Flag Printables: Accessed April 6, 2015,
   http://www.activityvillage.co.uk/iceland-flag-printables
Iceland Map: Accessed April 6, 2015, http://d-
   maps.com/pays.php?num_pay=199&lang=en.

Travel

Distance

From New York, NY, to Reykjavik is 2,617 miles. Flight time is 5 hours 44 minutes.

From Chicago, IL, to Reykjavik is 2,960 miles. Flight time is 6 hours 25 minutes.

From Dallas, TX, to Reykjavik is 3,761 miles. Flight time is 8 hours 1 minute.

From Seattle, WA, to Reykjavik is 3,624 miles. Flight time is 7 hours 45 minutes.

Hotels

Black Pearl. Located in Reykjavik, it offers apartments with full kitchens including cutlery, porcelain, and glassware for eight people, as well as luxury bed linens and complimentary coffee capsules. Within walking distance to landmarks, museums, shops, and restaurants.

Castle House Luxury Apartments. Located in Reykjavik near the airport, it features kitchenettes, free WiFi, and airport shuttle service.

Fosshotel Lind. Located in Reykjavik, it features smoke-free rooms, wheelchair access, free breakfast, a multilingual staff, and a dry cleaning service.

Grand Hotel Reykjavik. It features wheelchair-adapted rooms, a hot tub, spa, fitness center, on-site restaurant, lounge, and free breakfast.

Hotel Leifur Eiriksson. Located in Reykjavik opposite Hallgrims Church. It offers wheelchair access, an onsite bar, laundry services, and free breakfast.

Landmarks

Blue Lagoon. A man-made geothermal spa with crystal-clear water. The only place on earth where visitors can swim in 40-degree C water year-round, surrounded by ice and snow. The water is heated by the Svartsengi geothermal power plant.

Great Geyser. Located in southwestern Iceland, it has been active for over 10,000 years. It can spurt boiling water up to 70 meters in the air.

Gullfoss. Located near Reykjavik, it is called the Golden Circle because of amazing waterfalls and rock formations. When weather permits, visitors can see rainbows arching over the landscape.

Lake Myvatn. Here visitors can see the Waterfall of the Gods, the most famous waterfall in Europe, as well as bird life, volcanic craters, and lakes. In 1974 it was designated a protected conservation area.

Latrabjarg. An area of massive sea cliffs on Iceland's western shore, home to many types of birds, such as puffins, and providing an incredible view of the sea.

Raufarholshellir. A ¾-mile long underground cavern formed by ancient volcano lava tubes. Visitors can see unique ice candles and lava formations.

Travel Trivia

What does Reykjavik mean?
Smoky Bay.

True or false: Icelanders buy the most books in the world.
True. The Iceland literacy rate is 99 percent; the highest in the world.

How much of Iceland is useable for farming?
Only about one percent.

How much of the country has vegetation?
About a quarter. Only one percent of that land area is covered in trees.

True or false: Iceland is the most sparsely populated country in Europe.
True.

What are some animals native to Iceland?
Fox, mink, rats, rabbits, polar bears, and whales.

How much of Iceland is covered in ice and glaciers?
About 7,000 square miles.

Does Iceland have an army?
No. It is the only NATO country without armed forces.

True or false: Iceland has the highest life expectancy in the world?
True. 81.3 years for women and 76.4 years for men.

What is the main business in the country?
Fishing.

True or false: About 50 percent of Iceland's energy is geothermal.
True.

How many public pools are heated by volcanic water?
150.

True or false: Icelanders do not drink soda.
False: The country's residents drink the most Coca-Cola of anywhere in the world.

What must visitors do before entering a public pool?
Take a shower in a public area.

What is the highest point in Iceland?
The peak Hvannadalshnukur, at 2,110 meters.

What is Vatnajokull?
A glacier in Southeast Iceland which is Europe's largest glacier.

What is Hekla?
Iceland's most active volcano.

True or false: In 1963 a new volcano appeared in the Atlantic Ocean near Iceland and became the island of Surtsey.
True.

True or false: The Iceland phone book contains only first names.
True. Everyone is listed by first names only.

When can you see the Northern Lights?
The Aurora Borealis can be seen most reliably on clear nights in November and December.

America's Roots

Who was Jon Olafsson?
An Icelander who petitioned US President Ulysses S. Grant to form a colony on Kodiak Island in Alaska.

Who was Gunnar Hansen?
An actor famous for playing the character Leatherface in the movie *The Texas Chainsaw Massacre*. He was born in Iceland and moved to the United States at age 5.

Who was Leslie Stefanson?
An actress who starred in the movie *The General's Daughter*. She was born in Iceland.

Who was Leif Ericson?
An Icelandic explorer who many believe was the first to discover North America in 1000 AD.

Who were Thorarinn Haflidason Thorason and Gudmund Gudmundsson?
Icelanders who became Latter-Day Saints (Mormons) and settled in Utah in the 1850s.

Where in America did Icelanders settle during the late 1800s?
Milwaukee, Wisconsin.

Which US states had a high number of Icelandic immigrants?
Wisconsin, Minnesota, North Dakota, and Alaska.

What job did most Icelandic immigrants perform in America?
Farming.

What percentage of Icelanders moved to the United States in the twentieth century?
About 20 percent.

In the twenty-first century, what US state has the highest number of residents of Icelandic ancestry?
California.

When did the Icelandic National League form in the United States?
1919.

Who was Robert Samuel "Rob" Morris?
A professional linebacker for the Indianapolis Colts. His ancestors were from Iceland.

Who is Helgi Tomasson?
The artistic director and principal choreographer for the San Francisco Ballet and a former professional ballet dancer originally from Iceland.

Who is Aron Jóhannsson?
An American international soccer player who was born in Iceland.

True or false: American has the highest number of Icelander immigrants in the world?
False: The United States is second after Canada.

Sports and Games

Sports

Iceland has about 270,000 residents and, of that number, 15,000 play football, which Americans call soccer, the most popular sport in the country. There is a national association for football as well as a growing women's league for the sport, and many successful players travel to Europe and play professionally.

The most successful team sport is handball. About 10,000 Icelanders play and the country supports the sport with indoor courts and athletic houses. The men's handball league is considered one of the best in Europe.

Participation in golf has doubled over the last ten years, especially popular among children. There are about 5,000 active golf players and another 5,000 for whom golf is a hobby. The country supports the sport by adding and expanding golf courses.

Downhill and cross-country skiing are popular in Reykjavik where there are three ski areas even through extreme weather limits the sport to the months of January through March, though sometimes into the beginning of May. In addition, snowboarding is becoming a winter sport popular with young Icelanders, who use snowmobiles to visit the ice fields.

The warm Icelandic volcanic waters help to make swimming a very popular sport.

Sports Trivia

What is *glima*?
A form of wrestling popular in Iceland in which opponents throw each other by grabbing each another's belts.

True or false: Iceland hiking trails are marked in great detail.
False: Guideposts and markings are erratic. Hikers must be skilled with a map and compass.

What are the best months for hiking?
June through August has the best weather conditions.

What is Snaefellsjokull?

A dormant volcano that can be climbed. Novelist Jules Verne used it as the entrance to the earth in *Journey to the Center of the Earth.*

What is Vatnajokull?

A large ice cap and popular climbing spot.

True or false: There is whitewater rafting in Iceland.

True. It can be done on the rivers in the southwestern portion of the country.

True or false: There is no scuba diving in Iceland.

False: The country has clear waters and seal colonies that can be explored by scuba divers.

True or false: Vikings ate horses.

True. This practice was banned by Christianity.

True or false: Horseback riding is a popular sport in Iceland.

True. Riding ranges from day trips to two-week excursions.

What is Laugavegur?

A four-day long hiking trail through glaciers and valleys.

Game

Olsen Olsen is the Icelandic version of Crazy Eights.

Number of players: Two or more.

Materials. A standard deck of 52 cards.

To play. The dealer deals five cards to each player (seven each if there are only two players). The undealt cards are placed face down on the table, and the top card is turned face up. Starting with the player to the dealer's left and continuing clockwise, each player in turn must either place a card face up on top of the discard pile or draw a card from the undealt cards.

If the top card of the discard pile is not an eight, the player may play any card which matches the rank or suit of the previous card. For example, if the top card were the king of hearts, the player could play any king or any heart.

An eight may be played on any card, and the player of the eight must name a suit. If an eight is on top of the pile, the next player must play either another eight or any card of the suit named by the person who played the eight.

Winner. The first player who gets rid of all their cards wins and yells, "Olsen Olsen!"

ICHI benefits. Mental functions of language, speech, articulation, control of voluntary movement, muscle force, and mobility of joints.

Music and Dance

Music

The geography of Iceland has influenced its music. Due to its isolation, the music styles of the Middle Ages dominated into the nineteenth century. Instrumental music was non-existent and it was not until midway through the nineteenth century that part choral singing came to the island.

The arrival of new outside music spurred a rapid growth of musical ideas and talents. Icelander Jon Leifs became an internationally known classical composer and the Iceland Symphonic Orchestra was formed in 1950.

In the 1980s, Iceland was known for artists such as Sugarcubes and Sigur Ros. This continues with contemporary groups Gus Gus and Mugison.

The country hosts many musical festivals each year including the Techonics Festival, Reykjavik Artfest, and Sequences Real Time Art Festival.

Music Videos

#8 Miguson — Mur Mur: Accessed April 6, 2015,
   https://www.youtube.com/watch?v=THm5_m2Hs7Y
Apparat Organ Quartet — Romantika: Accessed April 6, 2015,
   https://www.youtube.com/watch?v=uynQmiXLaWo
Best Iceland Music: Accessed April 7, 2015,
   https://www.youtube.com/user/Besticelandicmusic
Iceland Music. Sigur Ros — Hljomalind: Accessed April 7, 2015,
   https://www.youtube.com/watch?v=wXCUOqQZ7nE

Dance

Traditional story-telling *vikivaki* dance has a long history in Iceland. In 1947 a group of young women brought ballet to the country and formed the Icelandic Association of Professional Dancers.

The first state-supported school for dance was established in 1952. It was not until 1973 that the first and only National Theater of Iceland and the Iceland Dance Company was formed.

Even after a late start, Iceland produces ballet of a quality recognized on the world stage. Icelander Helgi Tomasson was principal dancer for the New York Ballet Company for 15 years and later director of the San Francisco Ballet Company.

The first Reykjavik Dance Festival was held in 2002. This led to small dance groups being formed around the country.

Dance Videos

Dance Iceland: Accessed April 7, 2015,
    https://www.youtube.com/watch?v=VDdsHNq_V60
Iceland Dance: Accessed April 7, 2015,
    https://www.youtube.com/watch?v=Sk7arrJfTDQ
Icelandic Folk Dance: Accessed April 7, 2015,
    https://www.youtube.com/watch?v=2Mi1humhxAY

Music and Dance Trivia

Who is Helena Jonsodottir?
A choreographer and filmmaker who created the dance Open Source.

What is Mezzoforte?
Iceland's best known jazz group.

Who is Bjork?
A popular singer and member of the music band Sugarcubes.

Is there opera in Iceland?
Yes. The Icelandic Opera produces two operas each year.

Who is Vikingur Olafsson?
An internationally known Icelandic pianist.

Who is Saeunn Porsteinsdotti?
An internationally performing Icelandic cellist.

Who is Daniel Biamason?
An Icelandic classical composer and conductor.

Who is Gardar Thor Cortez?
A tenor with the Icelandic Opera.

Who is Bjom Thoroddsen?
A famous Icelandic jazz musician.

What is Dark Music Days?
An Icelandic classical music festival.

Food

Seafood, potatoes, and lamb are the mainstays of the menu in Iceland. Many other foods in Iceland are different from almost anywhere in the world. The typical menu includes minke whale, *skyr*, and *pylsur*, a type of hot dog.

Minke whale is not considered an endangered species. It is served in Iceland as kebabs or cooked the same as steak or tuna.

Skyr is a soft cheese that is similar to yogurt and is eaten daily in many forms.

Pylsur are made from lamb and a mix of pork and beef, and may include puffin meat. They are served on rolls and topped with *pylsusinnep*, a form of sweet brown mustard. Other popular toppings include ketchup, raw onions, and deep fried onions.

Other meats on the menu include lamb, reindeer steak, sheep's head, and fermented shark. The sheep's head is served on a plate with potatoes and mashed turnip. When feasting on sheep's head, diners are expected to eat the tongue, eyeballs, and ears but not the brain. *Lundi* is meat from puffins, small birds that live on the coastline of the country.

Icelandic snacks include *harofiskur* jerky which is wind-dried haddock layered in butter. Sweets include *ponnukokur*, a thin pancake served with jam or powdered sugar, and chocolate-covered licorice.

Recipe

Icelandic Torte. This treat is filled with prunes.
Ingredients.
For the cake:
1 cup butter
1 cup sugar
2 eggs
4 cups flour
2 teaspoons baking powder
¼ cup milk
1 teaspoon of vanilla
For the prune filling:
2 pounds dried prunes
1 cup sugar
½ teaspoon crushed cardamom seeds
¼ teaspoon salt
1 teaspoon vanilla extract

Preparation. Cream the butter and sugar together, Add eggs and beat well. Add the dry ingredients, milk, and vanilla. Chill the dough. Roll and cut into five parts. Roll each part into a circle and place on the bottom of a round cake pan. Bake at 350 degrees F. for 15 to 20 minutes.

Make the prune filling by finely chopping the prunes, then mix in all the ingredients except vanilla. Cook until the mixture is thick. Add the vanilla. Let cool.

After the torte bakes, add the prune filling between layers. Cover and store for one day before slicing and serving.

Food Trivia

What breads are popular?
Dark rye bread and rye flat bread.

True or false: Reindeer meat is served in restaurants.
True.

What is hakarl?
Shark meat.

True or false: Skyr is high in fat.
False: It is low fat.

What types of dried fish are popular?
Haddock, cod, and catfish.

What is *lax*?
Salmon.

What is *porrablot*?
The name of a mid-winter feast.

What were the Cod Wars?
A series of confrontations in the 1950s and 1970s between the United Kingdom and Iceland regarding fishing rights in the North Atlantic Ocean.

How did the Cod Wars end?
In 1976 the United Kingdom accepted a 200-nautical-mile fishing zone exclusive to Iceland.

How is lamb smoked in Iceland?
Over a fire fueled by birch wood or dried sheep dung.

Customs

Weddings

Icelandic engagements take time. The average length of an engagement is three to four years. The engagement is traditionally announced at least three separate times in a church. This is similar to the Catholic reading of the banns three times prior to a marriage in the church.

Once the wedding date arrives, a whole week of traditional gatherings, events, and celebrations occur. The day before the wedding the families of the bride and groom enjoy a party with food, drink, and toasts to the couple and to the Virgin Mary, the Mother of Jesus Christ. Guests are expected to entertain each other by singing songs and reciting poems.

A traditional church wedding is held on a Sunday. The groom and his party arrive first and when he arrives the church bells are rung signaling the bride that it is time for her arrival at church.

The bride enters the church with her bridesmaids and with a toastmaster who leads her to her groom. The wedding dress can be a traditional costume or, as has become more popular, a Western-style white gown with the groom wearing a tuxedo.

Children

Ancient legend requires that nine nights after birth, the child must be recognized by the father of the household by placing the child on his knee while sitting in the high seat. Water was sprinkled on the child, and then the child was named and admitted into the family. In the past, children were often named after deceased ancestors.

Holidays

January 1. New Year's Day
Variable date. Easter
Variable date. Easter Monday
April 23. First day of summer
Variable date. Whit Monday, the day after Pentecost
Variable date in May. Labor Day
June 17. Iceland Republic Day
December 25. Christmas
December 26. Second Day of Christmas
December 31. New Year's Eve

Customs Trivia

True or false: In Icelandic tradition, after the wedding reception the bride is undressed by her bridesmaids and wears only her headdress when she next sees her groom.
True.

What does the groom do when he enters the honeymoon suite?
He exchanges gifts with his bride.

What happens after the couple get into the bridal bed?
When the couple is secure in the bed, a priest enters the room and gives a blessing.

What happens after the priest's blessing?
The newlyweds drink from special bridal cups.

What is the seating arrangement at Icelandic weddings?
Tradition requires a high table for the newlyweds, their fathers, the best man, and the priest who conducts the wedding ceremony.

Where do guests sit at the wedding?
They are assigned seats in order of their importance at the event.

What new tradition have couples added in the last 100 years?
A post-reception party that lasts into the next day.

What games are played at the wedding reception?
A teasing game for the bride and groom.

What meal is served at a reception hosted by wealthy families?
Several courses of main dishes.

What is served at the reception hosted by a family of modest means?
Cakes and breads prepared by the family.

More Resources

DVDs

Fire & Ice Iceland, DVD, www.travelvideostore, 2007.
Globe Trekker: Iceland and Greenland, download, Amazon Video, 2010.
Iceland Europe's Wild Gem, download, www.travelvideostore.com, 2006.
Iceland's Favorite Places, DVD, www.travelvideostore.com, 2009.
Nature Wonders Dimmuborgir Iceland, DVD,
    www.travelvideostore.com, 2007.

Books

Hancox, E. *Iceland, Defrosted.* (Silverwood Books, 2013).
Krakauer, J. and Roberts, D. *Iceland: Land of the Sagas.* (Villard, 1998).

Le Bas, T. *Iceland*. (Insight Guides, 2014).

Leffman, D. Eyewitness Top 10 Travel Guide: Iceland. (DK Publishing, 2014).

Presser, B. and Bain, C. *Iceland Travel Guide*. (Lonely Planet, 2013).

Websites

Flag of Iceland: Accessed April 7, 2015, http://icelandflag.facts.co/icelandflagof/icelandflag.php

Government of Iceland: Accessed April 7, 2015, http://www.government.is/

The Official Gateway to Iceland: Accessed April 7, 2015, http://www.iceland.is/

US Department of State: US Relations with Iceland: Accessed April 7, 2015, http://www.state.gov/r/pa/ei/bgn/3396.htm

Visit Iceland: Official tourism Information Site: Accessed April 7, 2015, http://www.visiticeland.com/plan-your-trip/map-of-iceland

Photos

Arctic Photo Reykjavik Photo Gallery: Accessed April 7, 2015, http://www.arcticphoto.is/

Iceland: 18 Photos of Mind Blowing Beauty: Accessed April 7, 2015, http://theplanetd.com/iceland-photos-mind-blowing-beauty/

Iceland in Pictures: Accessed April 7, 2015, http://icelandinpictures.com/

Iceland: Pictures: Accessed April 7, 2015, http://www.tripadvisor.com/LocationPhotos-g189952-Iceland.html

Your Shot Iceland: Accessed April 7, 2015, http://travel.nationalgeographic.com/travel/countries/your-iceland-photos/

References

10 Must See Natural Attractions in Iceland: Accessed April 6, 2015, http://www.escapehere.com/destination/10-must-see-natural-attractions-in-iceland/?utm_medium=cpc&utm_source=google&utm_campaign=EH_GGL_US_D ESK&utm_content=select&utm_term=iceland%20landmarks.

Best Hotels in Iceland: Accessed April 5, 2015, http://www.tripadvisor.com/Hotels-g189970-zff12-Reykjavik_Capital_Region-Hotels.html

Card Games in Iceland: Accessed April 6, 2015, http://www.pagat.com/national/iceland.html

Five Best and Worst Icelandic Foods: Accessed April 7, 2015, http://www.planiceland.com/5-best-and-5-worst-foods/

Geography of Iceland: Accessed April 5, 2015, https://en.wikipedia.org/wiki/Geography_of_Iceland

Icelander Literature Center. Dance. 2015, Accessed April 6, 2015, http://www.islit.is/en/art-and-culture-in-iceland/dance/

Iceland Facts: Accessed April 6, 2015, http://www.kids-world-travel-guide.com/iceland-facts.html

Icelandic Americans: Accessed April 6, 2015, https://en.wikipedia.org/wiki/Icelandic_Americans

Iceland Music: Accessed April 6, 2015, http://www.iceland.is/arts-culture/music/

Iceland Quick & Fun Facts: Accessed April 6, 2015, http://midatlantic.icelandair.com/destination/iceland-facts/

Iceland: Quick Facts: Accessed April 5, 2015, http://www.iceland.is/the-big-picture/quick-facts/

Iceland Sports and Outdoor Activities: Accessed April 6, 2015, http://www.roughguides.com/destinations/europe/iceland/sports-outdoor-activities/

Iceland Torte: Accessed April 7, 2015, http://www.cooks.com/recipe/3q50y6o8/icelandic-torte.html

Iceland Wedding Traditions: Accessed April 7, 2015, http://www.worldweddingtraditions.net/icelandic-wedding-traditions/

Interesting Facts about Iceland: Accessed April 6, 2015, http://lifestyle.iloveindia.com/lounge/facts-about-iceland-1876.html

Norse Rituals: Accessed April 7, 2015, https://en.wikipedia.org/wiki/Norse_ritualsIreland

Sports in Iceland: Accessed April 6, 2015, https://www.verslo.is/erlend_samskipti/comenius/Comenius/ALT/vetur9900/group1%5Cindex.htm

Ten Cool Facts about Iceland: Accessed April 6, 2015, http://listverse.com/2013/12/15/10-cool-facts-about-iceland/

Travelmath Iceland: Accessed April 5, 2015, http://www.travelmath.com/from/Seattle,+WA/to/Reykjavik,+Iceland

IRELAND

Basics

Geography

Ireland, the Emerald Isle, is located near Europe between latitude 51.5 and 55.5 degrees north, and longitude 5.5 to 10.5 degrees west. The temperature ranges from 50.7 degrees F as an average high to 47.8 degrees F. for an average low. In an average year it rains about 151 days on the east and southern coasts to 225 days in the west.

The country's location and climate gives it a vibrant green color due to grass cover that flourishes in the mild moist air. A country of rolling hills and rocky soil, the western seaboard has no trees. This landscape feature is due to strong winds that limit tree growth as well as extensive forest clear cutting in the seventeenth century.

The Irish are one people split between two countries. Ireland, located in the southern portion of the island, includes 26 counties with a total area of 70,282 square kilometers, home to a population of 4,670,976 (July 2011). Six of the nine counties of the original County of Ulster in the north make up Northern Ireland, which remains part of the United Kingdom and has a population of 1,799,400 (January 2012). In 1973 Ireland became a member of the European Union.

Language

Ireland's national language is Irish, but it is spoken as the everyday language only in the Gaeltacht (Irish-speaking) regions of Galway, Kerry, Cork, Mayo, Donegal, and Waterford. In all other parts of Ireland, English is the spoken language.

History

Archeologists believe that the first humans arrived in Ireland in 10,000 BC, during the Mesolithic or Middle Stone Age period. The first settlers probably arrived by foot after crossing a land bridge that existed at that time between Ireland and Scotland. These people were mainly hunters.

The first people settled in the area known as the Ceide Fields of County Mayo, an area of bog land which is the oldest enclosed landscape in Europe and was under continuous cultivation for centuries. Agriculture in this area stopped about 5,000 years ago.

The Celts arrived in Ireland about 600 BC and eventually denominated the culture. The Celtic language and culture united the population by 200 BC.

The first and only king of an united Ireland, Brian Boru, formed an army around 1000 AD. They lived in the hills of Munster from which they attacked Norse settlements. In 1002 AD, Boru took the title *Ard Ri* and claimed monarchy of the whole Gaelic race. He was murdered by the Vikings in 1014 AD.

In the winter of 1171 AD, Henry II of England brought his army across the Irish Sea. He seized control of the country at the wattle palace of Dublin. The English built castles in what they considered their Irish colony.

In 1801 Ireland officially became part of the United Kingdom. On Easter Monday in 1916 Irish Catholics began a rebellion in Dublin. The fighting raged on for weeks before British troops defeated the rebels, but this was not the end of the fighting. On January 21, 1919, a fight for Irish independence began between Irish rebels and British troops.

The fighting ended in 1922 when the British Parliament passed the Government of Ireland act. This act separated Ireland into two separate countries. One consisted of the six counties of Ulster and the other consisting of three counties of Ulster and 23 southern counties. The six Ulster counties with a majority of Protestants accepted the act and formed Northern Ireland.

Map and Flag

Irish Flag to Color: Accessed February 28, 2015,
   http://www.coloringcastle.com/pdfs/flags/flag-ireland-123.pdf

Country of Ireland Coloring Pages: Accessed February 28, 2015, http://www.coloring.ws/ireland.htm

Travel

Distance

From New York, NY, to Dublin, Ireland, is 3,187 miles. Flight time is 6 hours 52 minutes.

From Dallas, TX, to Dublin, Ireland, is 4,471 miles. Flight time is 9 hours 27 minutes.

From Seattle, WA to Dublin, Ireland is 4,536 miles. Flight time 9 hours 34 minutes.

From Chicago, IL to Dublin, Ireland is 3,671 miles. Flight time 7 hours 50 minutes.

Hotels

Donegal Manor. Located in Donegal, it features free daily breakfast, WiFi, an onsite restaurant, and babysitting.

Galway Bay Hotel. Beautiful rooms, a wine tasting every Monday and Wednesday evening, and ballroom dancing with live music every Sunday and Thursday night free for guests.

Irish Landmark Trust. A restored eigtheenth-century guest house in Dublin which features beautiful rooms decorated with antiques.

Number 31. A guest house in Dublin which is the city's most distinctive property and the former home of modernist architect Sam Stephenson, who successfully fused 1960s style with eighteenth-century grace. Each morning gourmet breakfasts including kippers, homemade breads, and granola are served in the home's conservatory.

The Glasshouse. Located in Silgo, it has a fitness center, a tennis court, a bar and lounge, and offers smoke-free rooms.

Landmarks

Blarney Stone. No visit to Ireland is complete without a trip to this famous historical site located in the village of Blarney. Robert the Bruce gave this block of stone to the Irish people in gratitude for their unwavering support during the 1314 battle of Bannockburn.

Glendalough. The name means Valley of the Two Lakes. Located in the Wicklow Mountains, it was founded by St. Kevin, a hermit monk. It features mountain trails, monastic ruins, and a cathedral which is the biggest building at Glendalough.

Newgrange. A passage tomb located near the River Boyne in County Meath, and home to prehistoric monuments dating to 3200 BC — 600 years older than the Giza Pyramids in Egypt and 1,000 years older than Stonehenge. Built as a home for cremated remains, Newgrange is a well-constructed passage covered by a large mound held by large kerbstones which are believed to be fairy mounds. The Newgrange chamber is a tri-spiral Celtic design, known as a megalithic symbol of the Irish.

Ring of Kerry. Known as the Iveragh Peninsula, it is a place of overwhelming natural beauty with grass, flowers, ocean, and one of the finest beaches in Europe. Home to sports including golf, hiking trails, cycling paths, water sports, and fishing. It is also a historic site that includes Iron Age forts, Ogham stones, and old monasteries.

Rock of Cashel. Known as "St. Patrick's Rock," it served as the seat of the kings of Munster before the Norman invasion. The structures date to the twelfth century and is said to be the place where St. Patrick converted the King of Munster in the fifth century AD.

St. Kevin's Cross. An ancient cross with a ring, located in Glendalough. The round tower is 30 meters high with a door about 3.5 meters from the ground. This was once used as a storehouse.

Skelling Michael. Known as Michael's Rock, this 230-meter-high site of a seventh-century Irish monastery shows how the monks lived in small beehive-style huts above cliff walls. Located on the coast of Country Kerry, it became a popular pilgrimage destination in the 1500s.

Travel Trivia

Why is green associated with St. Patrick's Day?
It is the color of spring.

Why is the shamrock the traditional symbol of Ireland?
St. Patrick used it as a symbol to explain the Christian belief in the Trinity of God — Father, Son, and Holy Spirit.

What job do leprechauns perform?
They are the official shoemakers of the fairy kingdom.

What is the national flower of Ireland?
Shamrocks are the national flower of Ireland and are picked on St. Patrick's Day and worn on the shoulder.

When was the first St. Patrick's Day celebration in America?
In 1737, hosted by the Charitable Irish Society of Boston. The second celebration was established in 1780 by the Friendly Sons of St. Patrick in Philadelphia.

Where is Gaelic spoken?
Ireland, the Isle of Man, and in Scotland.

What is Irish coffee?
Hot coffee, Irish whiskey, and sugar, stirred together and topped with thick cream. The coffee is sipped through the cream.

Is Ireland the home of the potato?
No. The white potato, otherwise known as the Irish potato, originated in the Andean Mountains. In 1532 the Spanish arrived in north Peru and it is thought that they brought the potato to Europe in the second half of the sixteenth century.

What is the capital of Ireland?
Dublin.

What color is the Irish flag?
The national flag of Ireland, adopted in 1919, is a vertical tri-color of green (at the hoist), white, and orange. The Irish government has described the meaning behind each color: green represents the Gaelic tradition of Ireland, orange represents the followers of William of Orange in Ireland, and white represents peace, or a truce, between the Irish.

According to Irish legend, what does ringing in your ears mean?
A deceased friend is stuck in purgatory, the place sinners go before they can enter heaven, and is ringing a bell to ask for you to pray for him or her.

Who founded Dublin?
The Vikings, in 998 AD.

Why are the first three days in April called Borrowed Days?
This time is associated with bad weather that did not kill a cow. Legend says that March borrowed three days of terrible weather from April in a second attempt to kill the cow.

What is the oldest occupied castle in Northern Ireland?
Killyleagh Castle in County Down was built in the thirteenth century and is still in use as a private home.

Where was the first Irish constitution signed?
The Shelbourne Hotel in Dublin.

In olden days which member of the family farm was referred to as the gentleman who pays the rent?
A pig.

What is keening?
The Irish term for loud wailing, crying, and expressing love for the deceased at funerals.

What was Saint Patrick's real name?
Historians believe it was Maewyn Succat.

Who is the first saint of Ireland?
Saint Abban, who left Ireland to preach in England during the second century.

Who were the Children of Lir?
In an ancient Irish legend their wicked stepmother turned them into swans, but the swan-children kept their human voices and their singing brought 300 years of peace to Ireland.

America's Irish Roots

What city has the largest number of Americans of Irish descent?
Boston, with 23 percent.

How many US residents are of Irish descent?
34.5 million Americans claim Irish ancestry, which is nine times the current population of Ireland.

Who created the Oscar?
It was handcrafted by an Irishman, Cedric Gibbons, who was born in Dublin in 1823.

What Irish holiday is celebrated in the US by sending cards?
Over eight million St. Patrick's Day cards are exchanged in America, making it the ninth-largest card-selling occasion in the US.

How many American presidents had Irish ancestors?
Over 40 percent, including John F. Kennedy.

Who was Mike Quill?
Born in 1905 in County Kerry, Ireland, he was the founding president of the Transport Workers Union of America. During his tenure the US labor movement made great strides.

Who was St. Brendan?
An Irish monk who was a fifth-century sailor and may have discovered America before Christopher Columbus.

Who was Eamon De Valera?
The first President of the Irish Republic, born in Manhattan, New York City.

Who was James Hoban?
The Kilkenny-born architect who designed the original US White House in 1792 after winning a competition sponsored by President George Washington and Secretary of State Thomas Jefferson. When the White House was burned by the British during the war of 1812, Hoban oversaw the restoration of the building.

Who composed the melody of the *Star Spangled Banner*?
The blind Irish harpist Turlough O'Carolan.

Who was the first American general to die during the Revolution?
Donegal-born Richard Montgomery.

How is Muhammad Ali connected to Ireland?
His great-grandfather was born in Ennis, County Clare, immigrated to Kentucky in the 1860s, and married an African-American woman.

How is Walt Disney connected to Ireland?
He was born in 1901 in Hermosa, Illinois to an Irish-Canadian father and a German-American mother. He and his brother Roy co-founded Walt

Disney Productions. He won 22 Academy Awards during his lifetime and was the founder of the theme parks Disneyland and Walt Disney World.

How is George Clooney connected to Ireland?
His paternal great-great-grandparents Nicholas Clooney and Bridget Byron immigrated to the US from Ireland. He is an American actor, film director, producer, and screenwriter who has received three Golden Globe Awards and an Academy Award.

Who is Michael Ryan Flatley?
Born to Irish parents in Chicago in 1958, he is known for *Riverdance, Lord of the Dance, Feet of Flames*, and *Celtic Tiger*. In 1988 he set a Guinness Book world record for a tapping speed of 28 taps per second.

Sports and Games

Sports

The most popular sport in Ireland is Gaelic football, a combination of rugby, soccer, and American football. Players advance the football by carrying, bouncing, kicking, hand-passing, and soloing — dropping the ball and then toe-kicking it back into the hands. Neither players nor coaches receive payment for Gaelic football.

Coming in as second most popular is hurling, an outdoor sport that has been played for over 3,000 years and is becoming one of the fastest-growing team sports throughout the world.

In hurling, players use a wooden stick called a *hurley* to hit a small ball between their opponents' goalposts. The ball can be caught but carried for no more than four steps. It can also be struck in the air or on the ground with the *hurley* just as in field hockey. The ball can also be toe-kicked or slapped with an open hand for short-range passing. If a player wants to carry the ball for more than four steps he must bounce or balance the ball on the edge of the stick but only twice per possession.

Both Gaelic football and hurling have two 35-minute halves with a running clock which only stops in the event of injury or an on-field dispute.

Other sports popular in Ireland include golf, rugby union, cycling, cricket, rowing, netball, horse racing, show jumping, basketball, fishing, handball, target shooting, tennis, greyhound racing, boxing, and soccer.

Sports Trivia

How did hurling begin as an Irish sport?
Irish legend says that the warrior Cú Chulainn and other heroes created and excelled at hurling.

How popular is Gaelic football?
The most popular sport in Ireland with major games attracting 80,000 fans.

Who is Stephen Roche?
A famous cyclist born in Dundrum, Ireland, in 1959 and winner of the Road Race World Championship.

Who are the Shamrock Rovers?
An Irish football (soccer, to Americans) team established in 1901 and the most successful team in the country. They won 16 leagues of Ireland, 24 cups of Ireland, and 18 Leagues of Ireland Shield competitions.

What is the hurling ball called?
Sliotar.

What is the All-Ireland Final?
The premier Gaelic football competition, as important in Ireland as the American Superbowl.

Who is Shane Lowry?
A professional Irish golfer who won three Irish Opens.

True or False: Rugby was invented in Ireland.
False: It began in Great Britain in 1823.

What is another name for the Irish Football League?
The Airtricity League.

Do hurling players wear their names on their uniforms?
There are no names on the uniforms and the players' numbers are determined by their position on the field.

Game

Snap. A popular Irish card game.
Number of players. Two to 12.
Materials. A regular 52 card deck with the jokers removed.
To play. Cards are dealt face down with an equal number for each player. The first player places a card in the center of the table. This continues with each player placing a card on top of the last player's card. When a card placed on top matches the card below, such as a queen on a queen, the first person to yell "Snap" and hit the pile of cards with their hand wins all the cards. The game resumes with all players and remaining cards until one person has all the cards.
Winner. The first player to win all the cards.
ICHI benefits. Mental functions of language, speech, articulation, control of voluntary movement, and mobility of joints.

Music and Dan

Dance

Ancient Irish myths tell of harps that could kill men through the power of their music. The high kings of Ireland had their own personal harpists.

Throughout the centuries Irish folk music has told tales of battles won and lost. A song well known to many Americans, *When Johnny Comes Marching Home*, was written by the Irish during the Napoleonic Wars.

The failed Irish rebellion against the English in 1798 led to the composing of the songs *The Last Rose of Summer* and *The Minstrel Boy*.

The Irish who moved to America brought their love of country with them in songs such as *Galway Bay* and *Little Old House in the Oul Country Down*.

A famous Irish folk song is *Molly Malone,* also known as *Cockles and Mussels* or *In Dublin's Fair City*. The song, set in Dublin, Ireland, has become the unofficial anthem of Dublin City. It tells the tale of a fictional beautiful girl who worked as a fishmonger on the streets of Dublin but who died young of a fever in the seventeenth century. Its music and lyrics were written by James Yorkston:

In Dublin's Fair City
Where the girls are so pretty
I first set my eyes on sweet Molly Malone
As she wheel'd her wheel barrow
Through streets broad and narrow
Crying cockles and mussels alive, alive o!

The song was published in 1790 in Doncaster and later reprinted in 1831 in a collection entitled *The Shamrock: A Collection of Irish Songs.*

Music Videos

Relaxing Celtic Music — Spring Charm: Accessed April 5, 2015,
    https://www.youtube.com/watch?v=YGkuJlEZy04
The Chieftains: Accessed February 28, 2015,
    https://www.youtube.com/watch?v=1OuFWhA7FWg
The Dubliners performing Molly Malone: Accessed February 28, 2015,
    http://www.youtube.com/watch?v=diUkiTs1gxM
Two Hours of Celtic Music: Accessed April 5, 2015,
    https://www.youtube.com/watch?v=jiwuQ6UHMQg

Dance

The Irish jig is a compound-meter dance performed in 6/8 or 9/8 rhythm and part of Irish culture since about the seventeenth century. The word jig comes from the French word *gigue* and the Italian word *giga*, both of which mean to jump. The dance itself came from England and Scotland. Irish jigs were often danced in a competitive manner, where the winning dancer was the one who could dance the liveliest jig for the longest amount of time.

Irish dancers keep their hands at their sides when dancing. This practice dates back to when Ireland was under complete British control. Dancing was outlawed by conquering Normans in the twelfth century. Legend says that the Irish refused to give up dancing and adapted their dances by keeping their arms still so that whenever the English would look in the Irish people's windows, all they would see was a person with their hands at their sides. Thus their feet and legs were moving under the protection of the windows to conceal their outlawed dancing.

The Irish who immigrated to America in the 1700s brought their music and dance traditions to their new country. The Irish jigs and reels mixed with the bluegrass styles of the Appalachian Mountains.

Dance Videos

2½ Hours of the Best Celtic Music: Accessed April 5, 2015,
 https://www.youtube.com/watch?v=49En0xjh0Xg
Irish Dance Music: Accessed April 5, 2015,
 https://www.youtube.com/watch?v=yhvXfUxRkIg
Irish Dance World Championships Boston. 2013: Accessed February 28,
 2015, https://www.youtube.com/watch?v=gPylYGoquqM
Irish Dancing & Culture: Accessed February 28, 2015,
 http://www.irishdancing.com/
Riverdance: Accessed February 28, 2015,
 https://www.youtube.com/watch?v=HgGAzBDE454

Music and Dance Trivia

What famous classical composition was first performed in Dublin?
Handel's *Messiah* in 1742.

Who passed a law forbidding use of the harp?
Edward III, a Norman who ruled Ireland in 1366.

Who was Turlough Carolan?
An Irish harpist born in 1670 who wrote over 200 Irish tunes.

How did Irish harps differ from Welsh harps?
Irish harps had metal strings and Welsh harps had strings made of horse hair.

Who was George Petrie?
The publication of his book *The Ancient Music of Ireland* in 1895 ignited a folk music revival.

What song did Irish composer Harry Cohan write that every American knows by heart?
Yankee Doodle Dandy.

Name two popular Irish singing groups from the 1960s.
The Clancy Brothers and The Dubliners.

What movie made the song *Innisfree* famous?
The Quiet Man, starring John Wayne and Maureen O'Hara, which was written by John Farrell who, although never leaving Ireland, wrote this powerful song about leaving the Irish homeland.

Who organized the Irish band The Chieftains?
The Irish classical composer Sean O'Riarda.

Who wrote the words of the popular Irish song *Danny Boy*?
Historians believe the lyrics were written by English barrister Fred Weatherly.

What is an Irish couples' dance called?
A country set.

What is the name of Irish dances performed by a group of four, six, or eight dancers?
Ceili dances.

What instruments are traditionally used to play Irish dance music?
Fiddles, accordions, and flutes.

What rare Irish dance instrument resembles a Scottish bagpipe?
The Irish *uillean* pipe.

Who is Michael Flatley?
Irish dancer and founder of the popular dance show *Lord of the Dance*.

What instrument is prominent in the Irish dance performance *Riverdance*?
The drum.

When were Irish dancing hardshoes invented?
They were created in the seventeenth century by hammering nails into the soles of walking shoes.

How is a hardshoe different from a tap shoe?
The taps on a hardshoe are made of wood, fiberglass, or resin. Tap shoes have metal taps.

When do Irish dancers wear gillies?
These soft shoes made of leather are used by women for reel dances.

What are reelshoes?
A leather softshoe with a fiberglass heel that male dancers wear so they can click their heels together during the dance.

Food

When you ask what crop is grown in Ireland, the most common answer is potatoes, which is correct. Potatoes are served at almost every Irish meal. However, the Irish and Americans share other foods including onions, barley, sugar beets, wheat, and oats. Irish livestock includes sheep and cattle, grown for home use and for export. Fishermen for generations, the Irish use modern fish-farming methods and export fish.

Traditional Irish cooking is very basic with few ingredients because the people were very poor. Some favorite Irish meals, including *crubeens* (pigs trotters), tripe, and *drisheen* (a blood sausage), were all popular dishes and are still eaten in parts of the country. The Irish enjoy a fried breakfast which always includes pork sausages, bacon rashers, and black pudding, another form of blood sausage.

The most popular Irish dairy products are cheddar cheese and butter. The most popular bakery items are scones and Irish soda bread. Irish soda bread contains mainly flour, raisins, and caraway seeds.

Today a typical day's menu is bacon, eggs, and cereal for breakfast, meats and cheeses for lunch, and pork, beef, ham, or seafood for dinner.

Recipe

Scones. A popular Irish pastry, scones are said to be named for the Stone (or Scone) of Destiny, the place where Scottish kings were once crowned. Originally triangle-shaped, scones were made with oats and griddle-baked. Today's popular versions are flour-based, round, and baked in the oven. Makes about 8-10 small scones

Ingredients.
2 cups unbleached all-purpose flour
1 tablespoon baking powder
2 teaspoons granulated sugar
1 teaspoon salt
3 tablespoons unsalted butter, softened to room temperature

½ - ¾ cup milk, cream, or a combination

Preparation. Preheat oven to 350 degrees F. Place a baking sheet lined with parchment paper in the oven.

Sift together the flour, baking powder, sugar, and salt into a mixing bowl. With your hands work the butter into the dry ingredients until the mixture just holds together. Next, add ½ cup milk and mix until it forms into a soft, slightly sticky ball.

Place the dough on a very lightly floured work surface. Using a rolling pin, roll the dough to a 1" thick slab. Dip a 1" or 2" biscuit cutter in flour and cut out the individual scones.

Remove the baking sheet from the oven and arrange the scones on it. Bake for 8 minutes, then turn the sheet and bake another 4 minutes or until just barely brown.

To serve, top the scones with butter, preserves, or freshly whipped cream.

Food Trivia

Are potatoes native to Ireland?
No. They came to Ireland from South America in 1688.

What do the Irish call potatoes?
Praties.

What caused the potato famine?
In 1845 a fungus disease hit the Irish potato crop. The resulting famine killed millions of people.

What other crop is a basic food in Ireland?
Oats are a staple in the Irish diet, feeding not only the family but also livestock.

What foods are made with Irish oats?
Oatmeal porridge and oatmeal breads.

Name another food popular in Ireland.
Cabbage.

What fish are commonly eaten in Ireland?
Halibut, cod, trout, herring, salmon, and haddock.

What is the story of St. Patrick and whiskey?

St. Patrick was served less than a full measure of whiskey. He took this as an opportunity to teach the innkeeper a lesson about generosity. He told the innkeeper that a monstrous devil was living in the cellar of the inn, and that this devil fed on the dishonesty of the innkeeper. In order to banish the devil, the man must change his ways. When St. Patrick later returned, he found the bar owner generously filling the patrons' glasses to overflowing. St. Patrick returned to the cellar with the innkeeper, found the devil emaciated from the landlord's generosity, and promptly banished the demon, proclaiming thereafter everyone should have a drop of the hard stuff on his feast day.

What is *Pota Phadraig* or Patrick's Pot?

The custom of drowning the shamrock by floating a leaf of the plant in the whiskey before downing the shot.

Customs

Weddings

In a Christian ceremony, the couple light two candles and from these candles, light a third, a larger unity candle. The two original candles are blown out, showing that the two people are now one in unity.

Many superstitions are associated with weddings, including marry in white, everything's right, and a bride must wear something old, something new, something borrowed, something blue, plus an old Irish penny in her shoe.

Traditionally an Irish bride wears a garland of wild flowers, typically lavender, but modern brides wear a veil over their hair. In either case, a bride must never put her own veil or headdress on as this is considered very unlucky.

The traditional wedding ring is a *Claddagh* ring, molded gold showing two hands holding a crowned heart. It is very important when the ring is worn that the tips of the crown should be facing outward to indicate marriage. *Claddagh* rings were usually handed down from mothers to daughters for generations.

Fun traditional expressions associated with weddings include: to propose a groom to be might ask his future wife "Would you like to be buried with my people?" or "Would you like to hang your washing next to mine?"

Friends of a couple who want to know if a wedding is in the works may say, "When are you giving us a day out?" or "Should I buy a hat?"

Superstitions about marriage include tossing your hair into a bonfire to dream of your future mate and a mother-in-law should bake bread in the newly married couple's home to share her culinary skills.

Children

Superstitions associated with parenthood include a pregnant woman should not enter a graveyard because it would make her child weak and a pregnant woman should not be around rabbits or her child will have a hare lip.

Traditionally a pregnant woman should tie a string around her wedding ring and hold it over her stomach. If the ring moves in a circle the child is a boy, but a side-to-side swing means a girl.

An Irish father should sing to his child to form a bond before and after birth.

There are also health-related superstitions. To reduce the pain of labor, a friend should attach a broken needle to the pregnant woman's clothing.

Mothers are told to never eat an onion while nursing a child. It was thought that eating an onion would cause the child to be restless. Also, never rock an empty rocking chair or cradle as it will bring bad luck to the child.

When a child loses a tooth, the tooth should be buried in the yard so that a new tooth will grow in its place.

Celebrate the coming of age of a child by giving the child their own key to their house during their birthday party.

Holidays

January 1. New Year's Day
March 17. St. Patrick's Day
Variable date. Easter
Variable date. Easter Monday

First Monday in May. May Day
First Monday in June. June holiday
First Monday in August. August holiday
Last Monday in October. October holiday
December 25. Christmas
December 26. St. Stephen's Day
December 31. New Year's Eve

Customs Trivia

What is an old Irish birthday tradition for children?
The family lifts the birthday child, hold him/her upside down and give them a few gentle tap on the head, one for each year and one for good luck.

What's an ancient Irish cure for a hangover?
To be buried up to the neck in moist river sand.

What was an unusual Irish wedding custom?
Couples in Ireland could marry legally on St. Brigid's Day (February 1) in Teltown, County Meath, as recently as the 1920s by simply walking towards each other. If the marriage failed, they could divorce by walking away from each other at the same spot on St. Brigid's day the following year.

What is a pet day?
A single day of good weather that pops up in the midst of a long stretch of bad days.

What is cemetery Sunday?
A Sunday on which a Mass is celebrated for families with loved ones buried in the church graveyard. Family members clean their relatives' gravesite and everyone works together to clean the graves of the deceased who have no living relatives to care for their final resting place.

What does the saying "not backwards in coming forwards" mean?
A person who is not shy.

What does "no flies on him" mean?
A person who is not easily deceived.

What does "she has a tongue that would clip a hedge" mean?
A person who gossips.

What does "come for a day and stay for a week" mean?
Someone who outstayed their welcome.

What does "drown the shamrock" mean?
To put a few shamrocks into a glass and cover them with whiskey.

More Resources

DVDs

Come West Along the Road: Irish Traditional Music, DVD, Standing Room Only, 2007.
Discovering Ireland, DVD, Questar, 2001.
In Search of Ancient Ireland, DVD, PBS, 2002.
Passport to England, Ireland, and Scotland, DVD, Travel Channel, 2004.
Story of Ireland, DVD, BBC, 2002.
Visions of Ireland, DVD, Acorn Media, 2008.

Books

Campbell, K. *United Kingdom in Pictures.* (Lerner Publications, 2004).
Fitz-Simon, C. and Palmer, H. *The Most Beautiful Villages of Ireland.* (Thames & Hudson, 2011).
Hallowell, T. and Bell, K. *The Everything Travel Guide to Ireland From Dublin to Galway and Cork to Donegal: a Complete Guide to the Emerald Isle.* (Everything History & Travel, 2010).
Linton, E. *About Ireland.* (Forgotten Books, 2015).
Sullivan, R. *The Great Little Book of Fun Things You Probably Don't Know About Ireland.* (BookSurge Publishing, 2009).
Winn, C. *I Never Knew That About Ireland.* (Thomas Dunne Books, 2007).

Websites

Flag of Ireland: Accessed April 5, 2015, https://flagspot.net/flags/ie.html

Map of Ireland: Accessed April 5, 2015,
　　http://www.mapsofworld.com/ireland/
Ireland: Discover the Drama: Accessed July 20, 2012,
　　http://www.discoverireland.com/us/?WT.srch=1&WT.mc_id=us_ga_
　　010112_USGoogleAdwords_TI_US_B_Generic_Exact
The Government of Ireland: Accessed July 20, 2012, http://www.ireland-
　　information.com/reference/congov.htm

Photos

Ireland Tourist Bureau: Accessed July 20, 2012, http://away.com/travel-
　　gd-ireland-travel-photo-gallery-
　　sidwcmdev_094016.html?type=nopopup&gclid=CIDfo-
　　qW2rACFQrf4Aodbi1b0w
Royalty Free, Public Domain, Stock Photos: Accessed July 20, 2012,
　　http://pdphoto.org/PictureHome.php?cid=23&mat=pdef&md=cid

References

Agriculture Ireland: Accessed June 14, 2012,
　　http://www.nationsencyclopedia.com/Europe/Ireland-
　　agriculture.html#ixzz1yuaGgfq9
An Outline of the Geography of Ireland: Accessed June 16, 2012, http://www.ireland-
　　information.com/reference/geog.html
Best Places to Stay in Dublin: Accessed February 28, 2015,
　　http://www.lonelyplanet.com/ireland/dublin/hotels/best-places-to-stay-in-dublin
Birthday Traditions, Customs and Celebrations: Accessed June 14, 2012,
　　http://www.send-great-flowers.com/birthday- traditions.html#ireland
Brian Boru High King of Ireland. Accessed June 16, 2012.
　　http://limerick.com/history/brianboru.html
Ciaran Hinds Biography: Accessed June 26, 2012,
　　http://www.biography.com/people/ciaran-hinds-215221
Coming of Christianity to Ireland, St. Patrick: Accessed June 16, 2012,
　　http://www.wesleyjohnson.com/users/ireland/past/pre_norman_history/christianity.h
　　tml
Flag of Ireland: Accessed July 20, 2012, http://www.united-states-
　　flag.com/ireland3x5p.html# - Ireland flag
George Best Biography: Accessed June 26, 2012,
　　http://www.biography.com/people/george-best-9211159
History of Irish Music: Accessed February 28, 2015,
　　http://www.oracleireland.com/Ireland/history/irish-music.htm

History of the Irish Jig: Accessed June 23, 2012,
http://www.ehow.com/facts_4895096_history-irish-jig.html

Invasions of Ireland from 1170–1320: Accessed June 16, 2012,
http://bbc.co.uk/history/bristish/middle_ages/ireland_invasion_01.shtml

Ireland Famous Landmarks, Tourist Attractions & Best Places to Visit: Accessed June
16, 2012, http://famouswonders.com/europe/ireland

Ireland's Most Popular Sport. Not What You Think: Accessed February 28, 2015,
http://mtstandard.com/sports/ireland-s-national-sport-not-what-you-
think/article_a5e410d6-ad8d-11e3-8712-0019bb2963f4.html

Ireland's Scientific Heritage: Accessed June 26, 2012,
http://understandingscience.ucc.ie/pages/irish/scientists.htm

Ireland Superstition and Folklore: Accessed June 14, 2012,
http://www.atozworldculture.com/a-
z_culture_sample_content.asp?nid=20.34&cid=71&ada=y&parent=Culture

Irish Dance Facts: Accessed February 28, 2015, http://www.scott-
ellis.com/irishdancefacts.htm

Irish Food History: Accessed March 7, 2015,
http://homecooking.about.com/od/foodhistory/a/irishfoodhistry.htm

Irish Sayings: Accessed June 17, 2012, http://blog.goireland.com

Irish Timeline and History. 2012. A Timeline of Irish History: Accessed June 16, 2012.
http://rootsweb.ancestry.com/~fianna/history/

Irish Trivia: Accessed June 17, 2012, http://www.totacc.com/user/jornada/itrivia.htm

Map of Ireland: Accessed July 20, 2012, http://www.discoverireland.com/us/ireland-
places-to-go/explore-by-
map/?WT.srch=1&WT.mc_id=us_ga_010512_Maps_Display_Network

Music, Lyrics and Midis for Traditional Drinking and Folk Songs: Accessed June 18,
2012, http://www.ireland- information.com/irishmusic/irishsongs-music-lyrics-
midis.htm

Real Irish Scones: Accessed June 18, 2012, http://thekitchen.com/real-irish-scones-
128074

Snap – Card Game Rules: Accessed June 23, 2012,
http://boardgames.about.com/od/cardgames/a/snap.htm

Sports Played in Ireland: Accessed February 28, 2015, http://luisgnarbona-
sportsplayedinireland.blogspot.com/

The Insiders Tour of Ireland: Accessed June 16, 2012, http://www.ireland-fun-
facts.com/ireland-facts.html

The Irish Potato Famine: The Blight Begins: Accessed June 16, 2012,
http://www.historyplace.com/worldhistory/famine/begins.htm

The Origins of Irish Music: Accessed June 18, 2012,
http://www.standingstones.com/emaoitm.html

Travelmath Ireland: Accessed February 28, 2015,
http://www.travelmath.com/from/Chicago,+IL/to/Dublin,+Ireland

Twenty-Five Card Games: Accessed June 16, 2012,
http://www.britannica.com/EBchecked/topic/1232991/twenty-five

Twenty-Five, Fifty-Five, One Hundred and Ten: Accessed June 18, 2012,
http://www.pagat.com/spoil/5/25.html

Walt Disney Biography: Accessed June 26, 2012,
http://www.biography.com/people/walt-disney-9275533

What is the history behind the tradition of the tooth fairy?: Accessed June 14, 2012, http://wiki.answers.com/Q/What_is_the_history_behind_the_tradition_of _tooth_fairy

Where did the Term Scone come from: Accessed June 16, 2012, http://www.kitchenproject.com/history/Scones.htm

LUXEMBOURG

Basics

Geography

Luxembourg is a landlocked nation in Western Europe located at the intersection of Belgium, France, and Germany. It is one of the smallest nations in the world with an area of 998 square miles, which makes it slightly smaller than the US state of Rhode Island. The Ardennes Mountains extend from Belgium into the northern section of Luxembourg. The rolling plateau of the fertile Bon Pays is in the south.

Language

The official language established by law in 1984 is Letzebuergesch.

History

Luxembourg's history began when the country, once part of Charlemagne's empire, became an independent state in 963 AD, but that didn't last. In the fourteenth century, the territory was made up of two parts: Walloon was spoken in the French area and Letzebuergesch in the German area.

French occupation in the seventeenth century and the return of French troops in the late eighteenth century promoted the use of French and allowed it to become an important language in the administration, even in the German-speaking areas. After the Treaty of London of 1839 and the dismemberment of the Grand Duchy, the territory of the new independent state lay entirely within the German zone.

The Treaty of London of 1839 gave the western part of Luxembourg to Belgium and the eastern part became autonomous in 1848 as a Grand Duchy. Germany occupied the country in World Wars I and II. Allied troops liberated Luxembourg in 1944. Luxembourg joined NATO in 1949.

Map and Flag

Flag to color: Accessed April 4, 2015, Maps of the world. 2015.
　　http://www.mapsofworld.com/flags/luxembourg-flag.html
Luxembourg Map Coloring Pages: Accessed April 4, 2015,
　　http://www.mapresources.com/media/catalog/product/L/U/LUX-XX-
　　934510_comp_3.jpg

Travel

Distance

From New York, NY, to Luxembourg is 3,774 miles. Flight time is 8 hours 3 minutes.

From Chicago, IL, to Luxembourg is 4,263 miles. Flight time is 9 hours 2 minutes.

From Dallas, TX, to Luxembourg is 5,063 miles. Flight time is 10 hours 38 minutes.

From Seattle, WA, to Luxembourg is 5,065 miles. Flight time is 10 hours 38 minutes.

Hotels

Hotel Carlton. Located in Luxembourg near the railroad station and the National Museum of History and Art. Each room has a tea and coffee maker.

Hotel Mon Plaisir. Located in Strassen, a small and independent town, which is still considered as a part of the city of Luxemburg. It is a non-smoking building.

Le Place d'Armes. Located in the heart of Luxemburg City, featuring Art Deco, Baroque, and contemporary décor. It offers 24-hour room service, dry cleaning service, and free breakfast daily.

Melia Luxembourg. Located at the center of the triangle-shaped Place de l'Europe across from the Luxemburg Congress Center and within walking distance of the European Court of Justice, the Court of First Instance, the Court of Auditors of the European Communities, the Secretariat-General of the European Parliament, the European Investment Bank, and the Translation Centre for the Bodies of the European Union.

Parc Hotel Alvisse. Located at the edge of Luxemburg in a green setting. It features a free pool and sauna, free breakfast, and an on-site massage service as well as tennis, jogging, and bowling facilities.

Landmarks

Aquatower Berdorf. Visitors can learn about drinking water and tour the 55-meter high tower. The view from the tower offers spectacular views of Berdorf and its surroundings.

Casemates du Bock. A part of the city's old fortifications and the only UNESCO World Heritage site in the country.

Palace of the Grand Dukes. Also known as Grand Ducal Palace, it is situated in Luxemburg city and is the official residence of the Luxembourg grand duke and the offices of the Grand Duchy. Built in the late sixteenth century, it is decorated in Renaissance style.

Natural History Museum. Located in the Grund quarter on the eastern bank of the Alzette River near the Neumünster Abbey. Its eight separate scientific sections cover natural sciences such as botany, geology, ecology, geophysics and astrophysics, vertebrate and invertebrate zoology, paleontology, and mineralogy.

Notre Dame Cathedral. A Gothic-style church which was built by Jesuits in 1613. It contains the tomb of John the Blind, king of Bohemia and count of Luxembourg from 1310 to 1346. Many of the members of the royal family and noted bishops are also buried here in the tomb.

Train 1900. A tourist steam train which connects Pétange to Fond-de-Gras and Rodange in about an eight-mile journey.

Travel Trivia

True or false: Luxembourg is the least populated country in the European Union.
True. It has about 465,000 residents.

True or false: Luxembourg is the smallest country in the world.
False: It is the twentieth smallest among 194 countries.

What language is taught in Luxembourg schools?
German.

What language is used for business?
French.

True or false: Luxembourg has the highest per capita income in the world.
True. About US$115,000 per person.

What free internet calling company is headquartered in Luxembourg?
Skype.

What other internet companies have European headquarters in Luxembourg?
Amazon, Paypal, and Rovi.

How many banks are in the country?
155.

What European talent contest has Luxembourg won five times?
Eurovision Song Contest.

True or false: Luxembourg has won the European Song Contest more times than any other country.
False: Ireland is the leader.

Luxembourg has the highest minimum salary in the world. What is it?
US$13.89 per hour, as of 2013.

What mineral resource does Luxembourg have?
Iron.

What is the oldest city in Luxembourg?
Ecternach, founded in the seventh century.

Where is the airport?
In Findel, which is also a major cargo hub.

What is the main attraction in Remich?
Walking tours of the vineyards.

Who was Robert Schuman?
A native son who proposed the plan for the European Community and the European Coal and Steel Company.

What is *The Family of Man*?
The largest collection of world photographs, including photos from 68 countries, housed in the Clerveaux Castle.

What tributary of the Rhine forms part of the border with Luxembourg?
The Moselle flows 314 miles through Luxembourg and Germany.

What is the main industry of the country?
Banking.

True or false: The RTL Group in Luxembourg is Europe's largest media company.
True. It owns 34 TV and 33 radio stations in 12 countries.

America's Roots

Who was Wilhelm von Knyphausen?
A general who commanded German troops assisting the English against the Colonies during the American Revolution. He was born in Luxembourg in 1716.

Who was Edward Steichen?
A photographer, artist, and curator who created the exhibit *The Family of Man* for the Museum of Modern Art in New York. Born in Luxembourg, he came to America in the early 1900s.

Who is Arno Joseph Mayer?
A Luxembourg-born American historian who specializes in modern Europe, diplomatic history, and the Holocaust, and is currently Dayton-Stockton Professor of History (Emeritus) at Princeton University. He came to America in 1940.

Who was Hugo Gernsback?
An inventor and science fiction writer who came to America in 1904. In his honor, the award presented at the annual World Science Fiction Convention is named the Hugo.

Who was Loretta Young?
An American actress born in Utah, her ancestors came from Luxembourg. Starting as a child actress, she had a long and varied career in film from 1917 to 1953. She won the 1948 Academy Award for best actress for her role in the 1947 film *The Farmer's Daughter*.

Who was John Dennis "Denny" Hastert?
The fifty-ninth Speaker of the United States House of Representatives, serving from 1999 to 2007. He represented Illinois's fourteenth congressional district for 20 years, 1987 to 2007. His ancestors came from Luxembourg.

Who is Vincent Paul Kartheiser?
An American actor best known for playing Connor in the TV series *Angel* and Pete Campbell in *Mad Men*. His ancestors came from Luxembourg.

Who was the Reverend Theodore Martin Hesburgh?
A priest of the Congregation of Holy Cross, he was president of the University of Notre Dame for 35 years. His ancestors came from Luxembourg.

Who was Paul Oscar Adolph Husting?
A member of the United States Senate from 1915 to 1917. He was born in Wisconsin and his father was born in Luxembourg.

Who was Richard Francis "Dick" Kneip?
The twenty-fifth Governor of the US state of South Dakota, from 1971 until 1978. His ancestors were from Luxembourg.

Who was Paul Christian Lauterbur?
An American chemist who shared the 2003 Nobel Prize in Physiology or Medicine with Peter Mansfield for work which made magnetic resonance imaging (MRI) possible. He was born in Ohio and his ancestors came from Luxembourg.

Who was Matthew Woll?
President of the International Photo-Engravers Union of North America from 1906 to 1929, an American Federation of Labor (AFL) vice-president from 1919 to 1955, and an AFL-CIO vice-president from 1955 to 1956. He was born in Luxembourg and came to America in 1890.

Who was John Lawrence May?
An American clergyman of the Roman Catholic Church. He served as Bishop of Mobile (1969–1980) and Archbishop of St. Louis (1980–1992). He was born in Illinois and had ancestors from Luxembourg.

Who was Nicholas Muller?
A US Representative from New York whose ancestors are from Luxembourg.

Who is Christine Marie "Chris" Evert?
Born in Florida with some Luxembourg ancestry, she was known as Chris Evert-Lloyd from 1979 to 1987. She was a US professional tennis player who was ranked for years as the best in the world. She won 18 Grand Slam singles championships and three doubles titles, and overall won 157 singles championships and 29 doubles titles.

Sports and Games

Sports

Although Luxembourg does not have a national sport, sporting activities are considered an important national and social activity, and about a quarter of the population are members of a registered sports federation.

Due to the country's flat terrain, cycling and hiking are both popular sports in Luxembourg. There are extensive national networks of cycling and hiking paths. The Parc Naturel de la Haute-Sûre also provides great opportunities for walking, mountain biking, and horse riding.

Golf is popular, with over 4,000 fully licensed members and six golf courses. Other sports include sky diving, go-kart racing, cross country skiing, ice skating, and paragliding.

Sports Trivia

What ages can go go-karting?
Ages 10 and older.

Where is the best place for horseback riding?
Haute-Sûre Lake.

Where can people go cross country skiing?
Weiswampach.

Where can you join a rock climbing club?
University of Luxembourg.

Is there yoga in Luxembourg?
Yes, at the university and in private lessons.

Who was Josy Barthel?
Luxembourg's sole Olympic gold medalist who won the men's 1500 meters at the 1952 Summer Olympics in Helsinki.

How many tennis clubs are in the country?
Fifty-three. The oldest was founded in 1902.

Is there a cricket organization?
Yes. Cricket is a minority sport in Luxembourg, played predominantly by the British community.

When did the national football team organize?
1911.

True or false: Luxembourg made its first appearance at the Summer Olympic Games in 1900.
True.

Game

Koekhappen is a party game (modified below for residents) in which a soft treat is attached to a thread. Players have to try to bite the treat off the thread while keeping their hands behind their backs. *Aappelhappen* is another version of the game in which an apple coated with maple syrup is attached to the thread. The syrup makes it more difficult to bite into the apple and the risk of being smeared by the syrup adds to the fun.

Number of players. The total players must be an even number.

Materials. Chocolate cookie dough, oven, and yarn. Bake soft chocolate chip cookies, enough for each participating resident. Put a pencil-sized hole in each one before baking. When the cookies are baked, string the yarn through the cookie hole.

To play: String soft cookies on a rope. Then pair up the residents. One resident holds the rope while the other eats a cookie off the string without using their hands. Then reverse the roles of holder and eater.

Winner. Whoever is fastest to successful eat a cookie.

ICHI benefits. Voluntary control of movements, joint mobility, and muscle force.

Music and Dance

Music

The history of music in Luxembourg goes back to the third century when citizens played the flute and the lyre.

Church music took center stage in the eighth century when the Abbey of Echternach became important. Around 900 AD, the Abbey produced the *Officium Sancti Willibrordi* manuscript, one of the first examples of musical notation from Luxembourg.

After Luxembourg was established in 1815, patriotic music and military bands increased interest in music throughout the country. In 1842 the Luxembourg Army Band, known as the Musique Militaire Grand-Ducale, was founded in Echternach with 25 musicians from the battalion.

In 1852 the Société Philharmonique was founded in Ettelbrück by Father J. B. Victor Müllendorf with the objective of supporting all types of vocal and instrumental music.

On the occasion of the first train from Luxembourg to Thionville in October 1859, the national poet Michel Lentz wrote the words and music for *De Feierwon*, a patriotic song which includes the famous line *mir welle bleiwe wat mir sin*, meaning *we want to remain as we are*.

Today citizens enjoy a wide range of music from classical to jazz and from rock to folk.

Music Videos

Luxembourg Music: Accessed April 4, 2015,
    https://www.youtube.com/watch?v=imwHjjcC_zs
Luxembourg music and images: Accessed April 4, 2015,
    https://www.youtube.com/watch?v=qURFlRadgbs
Luxembourg National Day 2013: Music by Monophona: Accessed April
    4, 2015, https://www.youtube.com/watch?v=8lO8Dk4jsc0
Luxembourg River Music: Accessed April 4, 2015,
    https://www.youtube.com/watch?v=yIGKN20NLcA
Music on the Street in Luxembourg: Accessed April 4, 2015,
    https://www.youtube.com/watch?v=clYxkxmzXyY

Dance

The dance of Luxembourg is *hopping*, a bouncy dance to the tune of a polka, in honor of the country's patron saint, St. Willibrord. Europe's largest traditional dancing procession is held annually on Whit Tuesday, the day before Ash Wednesday. It attracts 10,000 *hoppers* and 40,000 spectators to Echternach.

St. Willibrord was an Anglo-Saxon missionary from Ripon in North Yorkshire, England, who is credited with driving paganism out of Belgium, the Netherlands, and Germany during the eighth century. He is revered as a healer of epilepsy and nervous diseases.

The dance starts early in the morning in the courtyard of the abbey founded by Willibrord in 698 AD and slowly moves around the town. From toddlers to octogenarians with walking sticks, people form 45 groups, each containing rows of five dancers wearing simple white tops and black skirts or trousers.

Dancing begins when the marching band starts up a catchy polka tune, which is played over and over again until the procession ends a few hours later inside the abbey's crypt. Once a multi-step affair involving backwards jumps, the modern version of the dance is quite simple — a little jump to the right, a little jump to the left, and hop you go forward.

The dancers in each row hold on to a folded cloth to help synchronize the hopping. Hitler tried to stop the annual event but in 1941 a group secretly hopped inside the abbey to defy the Nazis. The day the Nazis left, the dance returned, accompanied by harmonicas and flutes. Luxembourgers danced through the rubble of the basilica which had been blown up by the Germans.

Dance Videos

Dance Luzembourg Hop Religious Procession: Accessed April 4, 2015,
   https://www.youtube.com/watch?v=YkwjJNttuWA
Levan Polkka Leekspin-Dance in Luzembourg: Accessed April 4, 2015,
   https://www.youtube.com/watch?v=T0pjiQYfR4U
Luzembourg's Annual Hopping Festival: Accessed April 4, 2015,
   http://www.bbc.com/news/magazine-23932767
Vligger. Luxembourg: Accessed April 4, 2015,
   https://www.youtube.com/watch?v=adQYZK0xIwk
Zornista in Luxembourg: Accessed April 4, 2015,
   https://www.youtube.com/watch?v=F5-jkqWMvBo

Music and Dance Trivia

What is the *UGDA*?
The Union Grand-Duc Adolphe (UGDA) is the national music federation.

What is the national anthem?
Ons Hémécht, meaning *our homeland*. In 1895 Jean-Antoine Zinnen wrote the music and Michel Lentz wrote the lyrics.

Who was Laurent Menager?
He is called Luxembourg's national composer. In 1857 he founded the national choral association Sang a Klang.

When was the Luxembourg Philharmonic Orchestra, originally known as the RTL Grand Symphony Orchestra, founded?
1933.

True or false: Opera is performed in Luxembourg.
True. In Luxembourg City at the Grand Théâtre, in Esch-sur-Alzette at the Théâtre d'Esch and at the annual Wiltz festival.

What is Kate?
A five-member indy-folk-pop group which started in 2008.

Who are Ernie Hammes and Gast Waltzing?
Jazz trumpet players.

Who is Sandrine Cantoreggi?
An internationally known violinist.

Who is Pascal Schumacher?
A jazz musician, composer, and percussionist who has founded a number of groups including the Pascal Schumacher Quartet.

How many students are enrolled in the Luxembourg Conservatory of Music?
About 2,600 students annually.

Food

Luxembourg food is a combination of French and German cuisine, with the cuisine of Italian and Portuguese immigrants added to the mix. Traditionally Luxembourgers eat a small breakfast and large meals at midday and in the evening.

Special foods are consumed on national and religious holidays, as well as on Sunday afternoons. After consuming these large meals, Luxembourgers are fond of taking walks in the country.

Specialties include *Judd matt Gaardebounen*, smoked collar of pork with broad beans, and *thuringer*, small sausages. Luxembourg ham is smoke-cured and *friture de la Moselle* is a small deep-fried river fish.

Other traditional favorites include potato pancakes, *kach keis* which is soft melted cheese, and *quetsche tort* which is plum tart.

Meals are served with dry white wine produced from Reisling grapes grown on the east-facing slopes by the Moselle River in Luxembourg. The country also produces plum brandies made from yellow and purple plums.

Recipe

Hot Potato Salad or *Warem Gromperenzallot* is many a Luxembourger's favorite dish. Serves about 20 residents for a tasting.

Ingredients.
4 pounds potatoes
2 ounces bacon fat
Salt and pepper
3 onions
1 tablespoons olive or salad oil
2 or 3 tablespoon butter
3 tablespoons vinegar
Parsley.

Preparation. Boil the potatoes in their jackets and peel while still hot. Cut the potatoes into slices and mix with the salt, pepper, oil, and vinegar. Keep the mixture warm. Cut the bacon fat into small cubes and fry. Pour the bacon over the hot potatoes and garnish with parsley.

Food Trivia

True or false: Jugged hare is a popular dish.
True.

True or false: Luxembourg sells the most alcohol in European GDP.
True.

Immigrants always bring new foods to a country. How many immigrants are there in Luxembourg?
As of 2006, there were 181,000 immigrants in Luxembourg, accounting for 39.6 percent of the total population. Fifteen percent of the country's inhabitants are of Portuguese origin.

Name some popular vegetables.
Lettuce, carrots, asparagus, cauliflower, broccoli, spinach, potatoes, and onions.

True or false: The country sells more prepackaged food now than in the past.
True, due to the high number of women in the work force.

What are some popular fruits?
Apples, oranges, pears, strawberries, peaches, bananas, apricots, and grapes.

What are some popular meats?
Chicken, beef, lamb, and pork.

Name other popular foods.
Milk, eggs, and honey.

What is *Äppelkuch*?
Apple pie.

What is *Boxemannercher* and when is it served?
A dessert served on St. Nicholas Day.

Customs

Weddings

Luxembourg has specific laws concerning marriage. The minimum age for marriage in Luxembourg is 18 years old. Minors need parental consent before they may marry.

Luxembourg law only recognizes civil marriage which must be performed by a Luxembourg civil registrar. Religious ceremonies are optional, have no legal status, and may only be held after the civil ceremony has taken place. It can, but need not, be on the same day.

Marriage rates have dropped sharply in recent years. One-third of couples who live together are unmarried, one-seventh of children are born to unmarried mothers, and one-third of marriages end in divorce. All these practices were rare a generation ago.

Children

Among native-born Luxembourgers, the birth of a baby is a relatively rare event at about 3,000 per year, several hundred less than the annual number of deaths. An extensive publicly supported network of day care centers is available for mothers who work outside the home. Nearly half the babies are born to foreigners, and they are entitled to the same maternity and day care as the native-born population.

Creativity and expressiveness are not emphasized in child rearing. An infant is not the constant center of attention, and parents are not obsessed with constant catering to a child's whims. Regular mealtimes and other activities are not disrupted by the arrival of a child.

Holidays

January 1. New Year's Day
Variable date. Easter
Variable date. Easter Monday
Variable date. Whit Monday, the day after Pentecost
Variable date in May. Labor Day
Variable date. Ascension
June 23. National Holiday
December 25. Christmas
December 26. St. Stephen's Day
December 31. New Year's Eve

Customs Trivia

Why do brides cut a wedding cake?
The tradition comes from ancient Rome, where revelers broke a loaf of bread over a bride's head for fertility's sake.

What happens if the younger of two sisters marries first?
The older sister must dance barefoot at the wedding or risk never landing a husband.

Why does the bride stand to the groom's left during a Christian ceremony?
In olden days the groom needed his right hand free to fight off other suitors.

Why did Catholics post wedding banns?
To announce an upcoming marriage to ensure the bride and groom were not related.

Why is the wedding cake tiered?
The custom of tiered cakes emerged from a game in which the bride and groom attempted to kiss over an ever-higher cake without knocking it over.

Why do brides carry or wear something old on their wedding day?
To symbolize continuity with the past.

Why do brides wear a veil?
Ancient Greeks and Romans thought the veil protected the bride from evil spirits.

What does the color aquamarine mean at a wedding?
It represents marital harmony.

Why is a pearl engagement ring bad luck?
Because its shape echoes that of a tear.

Where do most women wear their wedding ring?
Seventy percent wear their ring on the fourth finger of their left hand.

More Resources

DVDs

Belgium & Luxembourg, DVD, Globe Trekker, 2007.
Holland/Luxembourg/Belgium, DVD, Questar VHS, 1993.
Low Countries: Holland, Belgium & Luxembourg, DVD, Questar VHS, 2002.
Normandy, Belgium & Luxembourg, DVD, Small World Productions, 1993.
Railways of Belgium & Luxembourg, DVD, Artsmagic, 2014.

Books

Dunford, M. *The Rough Guide to Belgium and Luxembourg* (Rough Guides, 2015).

Elliott, M. and H. Smith. *Belgium & Luxembourg Travel Guide*, (Lonely Planet, 2013).

Skeleton, T. *Luxembourg*, (Bradt Travel Guide, 2012).

Tait, P., McPeake, L., Mason, A., and Colwell, D. *DK Eyewitness Travel Guide: Belgium and Luxembourg* (DK Publishing, 2013).

Websites

Flag of Luxembourg: Accessed April 5, 2015, www.worldflags101.com/l/luxembourg-flag.aspx

Government of Luxembourg: Accessed April 5, 2015, http://www.luxembourg.public.lu/en/

Grand Duchy of Luxembourg: Accessed April 5, 2015, http://www.visitluxembourg.com/en/what-to-do/arts-culture/sightseeing

Map of Luxembourg: Accessed April 5, 2015, http://www.mapsofworld.com/luxembourg/

US Embassy Luxembourg: Accessed April 5, 2015, https://www.facebook.com/usdos.Luxembourg

Photos

Luxembourg Photos: Accessed April 5, 2015, http://www.trekearth.com/gallery/Europe/Luxembourg/

Luxembourg Pictures: Accessed April 5, 2015, http://www.luxembourgpictures.com/

Luxembourg: Pictures: Accessed April 5, 2015, http://www.tripadvisor.com/LocationPhotos-g190340-Luxembourg.html

Pictures of Luxembourg and Clervaux: Accessed April 5, 2015, http://www.globetrotter.photography/luxembourg/luxembourg.html

Photogallery of Luxembourg: Accessed April 5, 2015, http://www.orangesmile.com/travelguide/luxembourg/photo-gallery.htm

References

74 Hotels in Luxembourg: Accessed April 4, 2015,
http://www.booking.com/city/lu/luxembourg.html

Boxemännercher: Accessed April 4, 2015,
http://recipes.wikia.com/wiki/Boxem%C3%A4nnercher

Countries and Their Cultures. Luxembourg: Accessed April 4, 2015,
http://www.everyculture.com/Ja-Ma/Luxembourg.html

Explore Your World. Luxembourg: Accessed April 4, 2015,
http://www.worldatlas.com/webimage/countrys/europe/luxembourg/lufamous.htm

Fun Trivia Luxembourg: Accessed April 4, 2015,
http://www.funtrivia.com/en/Geography/Luxembourg-4154.html

Hot Potato Salad: Accessed April 4, 2015,
http://www.alleasyrecipes.com/recipes/5/1/hot_potato_salad.asp

Interesting Facts about Luxembourg: Accessed April 4, 2015,
http://www.eupedia.com/luxembourg/trivia.shtml

Landmarks and Historic Sites. Luxembourg: Accessed April 4, 2015,
http://www.placesonline.com/europe/luxembourg/luxembourg/landmarks_and_histo
ric_sites/

Luxembourg: Accessed April 4, 2015,
http://www.infoplease.com/country/luxembourg.html?pageno=2

Luxembourg. Things to Do: Accessed April 4, 2015,
http://www.visitluxembourg.com/en/place/misc/train-1900-fond-de-gras

Sport in Luxembourg: Accessed April 4, 2015,
https://en.wikipedia.org/wiki/Sport_in_Luxembourg

Superstitions in Luzembourg: Accessed April 4, 2015,
http://www.bestcountryreports.com/Soci_Luxembourg_Superstitions_Folklore.php

Travelmath Luxembourg Accessed April 4, 2015,
http://www.travelmath.com/from/Seattle,+WA/to/Luxembourg,+Luxembourg

NETHERLANDS

Basics

Geography

The Netherlands is located on the coast of the North Sea and is part of the great plain of north and west Europe. Almost half the country's area is below sea level, making the famous Dutch dikes necessary for efficient land use. The water is drained into the North Sea and the principal rivers, the Rhine, Maas, and Schelde, which begin outside the country. The Netherlands is about twice the size of the US state of New Jersey.

Language

The official language is Dutch. The regional and minority languages are: Frisian, Low Saxon, and Limburgish.

History

Dutch history began with Celtic and Germanic tribes living in a harsh land geographically isolated from the rest of Europe. However, in 1 BC the Roman Empire conquered the southern part of the Netherlands and established a military post in Nijmegen. The Romans never investigated the northern areas of what would become The Netherlands and the southern areas remained under Roman control for about 300 years.

When the Roman Empire fell, more Germanic tribes arrived and the Franks invaded the territory in the fifth century and brought Christianity.

By 800 AD the Netherlands was a part of the powerful Frankish Empire of Charlemagne.

After the fall of the Frankish Empire with Charlemagne's death in 814 AD, the Low Countries area of the Netherlands was divided into several smaller states ruled by dukes and counts. At the same time, it became one of the richest areas in Europe due to agriculture, crafts, and commerce, trading as far as Asia and North Africa.

Political troubles began when the neighboring Dukes of Burgundy and the Habsburgs tried to dominate the Netherlands and introduce taxation. In 1555 Charles of the Habsburg dynasty granted the Netherlands to his son King Philip II of Spain. This began 80 years of fighting that fueled the national identity of the Netherlands. The country gained freedom from Spain in 1581, and in 1648 the Spanish recognized the sovereignty of the Republic. The Dutch Republic remained under the control of the Austrian throne of Habsburg until 1794.

During those years of war, the Dutch continued to travel the seas, discovering new routes and lands. By the mid-seventeenth century, the Republic was the biggest maritime power in Europe, and Amsterdam was the most important financial center on the continent. At the beginning of the eighteenth century, the domination of France, Austria, Russia, and Prussia on the continent, and the United Kingdom on the sea, led to the demise of the tiny Dutch Republic.

The eighteenth century saw the establishment of the Kingdom of the Netherlands which, after the fall of Napoleon, also included the territories of today's Belgium and Luxembourg. Belgium revolted and in 1830 became the Kingdom of Belgium. Luxembourg finally separated from the Kingdom of the Netherlands in 1890.

During World War I, the Netherlands remained neutral. During World War II, Germany invaded and occupied the Netherlands. After post-war reconstruction, the Netherlands made a rapid economic recovery and today is one of the most developed and wealthiest countries in the world.

Map and Flag

Country of Netherlands Coloring Page. Accessed April 3, 2015,
   http://www.coloring.ws/netherlands.htm

Netherlands Flag: Accessed April 3, 2015,
http://www.mapsofworld.com/flags/netherlands-flag.html

Travel

Distance

From New York, NY, to Amsterdam is 3,654 miles. Flight time is 7 hours 48 minutes.

From Chicago, IL, to Amsterdam is 4,119 miles. Flight time is 8 hours 44 minutes.

From Dallas, TX, to Amsterdam is 4,922 miles. Flight time is 10 hours 21 minutes.

From Seattle, WA, to Amsterdam is 4,879 miles. Flight time is 10 hours 15 minutes.

Hotels

B&B Helmers. Located in Amsterdam. It offers free WiFi, en suite bathrooms, fully stocked kitchenettes, Nespresso coffee machines, a flat-screen TV, and air conditioning. Guests can prepare their own breakfasts and, weather permitting, eat on the roof terrace.

CitizenM Hotel Amsterdam Airport. Located in Amsterdam. Perfect for a visitor's last or first night when location near the airport is a must. It features 24-hour food service, free WiFi, and LCD TVs with free movies. Each room is soundproofed and has blackout curtains, an oversized bed, a safe, and rainfall showerheads in the bathroom.

Grand Dutch Residence. Located in Amsterdam within walking distance of the Van Gogh Museum and the Royal Carre, it was built in 1867 and features the Michelin-starred restaurant La Rive overlooking the Amstel River. It also has crystal chandeliers and a heated indoor pool.

Hotel De Kastanjehof. Located in the Lage Vuursche forest, it features a beautiful garden with a large pond, a lovely terrace, and an enclosed backyard. Hotel visitors can view the Castle Drakestein.

InterContinental Amstel. Located in Amsterdam. Pets are allowed in the hotel rooms for an extra $65 per night. The staff speak both English and Dutch.

SS Rotterdam Hotel en Restaurants. Located in Rotterdam on the riverfront near the Erasmus Bridge in an anchored ship with hotel suites and restaurants on board. The deck features a shallow swimming pool.

Landmarks

Anne Frank House. Anne, a young Jewish girl, was forced into hiding with her family and their friends in Amsterdam to escape deportation by the Nazis. This house Otto Frank used as a hideaway for his family kept them safe until close to the end of World War II.

The focus of the Anne Frank House museum is the rear of the house, also known as the secret annex, which looks as it did during World War II. In this dark, airless space the Franks observed complete silence during the day and read Dickens before being mysteriously betrayed and sent to their deaths.

Central Grachtengordel Canal Belt. The best known of the three rings of Amsterdam canals, lined by elaborately decorated merchants' residences and warehouses built in the seventeenth century. Ninety islands were created when the canals were built, all connected by hundreds of charming bridges.

Hermitage Amsterdam. Located in Amsterdam. One of the largest museums in the country, its collections include Russian artifacts and nineteenth- and twentieth-century French paintings.

Keukenhof Gardens and Tulip Fields. Open from March to May. Visitors can see over seven million tulips, daffodils, hyacinths, and other spring bulbs in bloom. The fields cover 79 acres and are the world's largest garden.

Rijksmuseum (National Museum). The premier art museum of the Netherlands. The collection includes some 5,000 paintings, most importantly those by Dutch and Flemish masters from the fifteenth to nineteenth centuries. The museum also houses collections of sculpture, applied art, Dutch history, and Asiatic art, including the famous twelfth-century Dancing Shiva. The museum's print archives have over 800,000 prints and drawings.

Vincent Van Gogh Museum. Located in Amsterdam, the museum houses about 200 paintings and 500 drawings by Van Gogh and his friends and contemporaries, including Gauguin, Monet, Toulouse-Lautrec, and Bernard, as well as many of Van Gogh's personal effects.

Travel Trivia

True or false: The Netherlands and Holland are the same.
False: Holland is the western portion of the country.

True or false: The Schiphol Airport is below sea level.
True. The Dutch are experts at keeping out seawater.

What percentage of the world's flower bulbs come from the Netherlands?
Seventy-five percent.

What is the purpose of the Dutch windmills?
To pump away excess water.

What percentage of the residents speak English?
Eighty-six percent.

What city is the largest port in the world?
Rotterdam.

Why is Eindhoven called the City of Light?
The Phillips electronic company makes light bulbs in the city.

True or false: The Netherlands are the largest exporter of cheese in the world.
True.

How many museums are there in the Netherlands?
1,000.

Who was Rembrandt van Rijn?
A Dutch painter who became world famous for his work *The Night Watch*.

How many windmills are there in the Netherlands?
1,000 vertical windmills. There were originally 10,000.

When were wooden shoes invented to keep farmers' feet dry?
700 years ago.

True or false: The Dutch put ice cream sprinkles on their toast.
True.

True or false: The Netherlands are the bicycle capitol of the world.
There are over 18 million bikes, more than one per person.

How long have there been cheese markets in the Netherlands?
Over 300 years.

True or false: The Dutch people own the most umbrellas in the world.
False: The do not use umbrellas. They wear rain suits because the wind is too strong for an umbrella and it is also impossible to hold an umbrella and ride a bicycle.

What is the Dutch name for wooden shoes?
Klompen.

What is the most popular snack food?
French fries dipped in mayonnaise.

True or false: The Netherlands has the highest number of part-time workers in the European Union.
True. Four out of every ten workers are part time.

In what year was the Netherlands the first country in the world to legalize same-sex marriage?
2001.

America's Roots

Who was Bart Jan Bok?
A graduate of the University of Leiden's Astronomy Department and a naturalized American. In 1929 he accepted a position at Harvard University where he helped set up the National Observatory of Mexico at Tonantzintla and Harvard's southern station observatory in South Africa.

Who was James Van Hoften?
A US astronaut who flew on two NASA missions, the seven-day STS-41-C Challenger flight which took off on April 6, 1984, and the seven-day STS-51-I Discovery flight which took off on August 27, 1985. He is of Dutch ancestry.

Who was John Hasbrouck Van Vleck?
The first Dutch-American to be awarded the Nobel Prize in Physics, which he received in 1977 at age 78 for his contributions to the understanding of the behavior of electrons in magnetic solids. He is regarded as the founder of the modern quantum mechanical theory of magnetism.

Who was Peter Debye?
The first Dutch American to be awarded the Nobel Prize in Chemistry which he received in 1936 for his contributions to the study of molecular structure, primarily for his work on dipole moments and X-ray diffraction.

Who was Angelica Schuyler Church?
The oldest daughter of Continental Army General Philip Schuyler and Catharine Van Rensselaer Schuyler, she married British MP John Barker Church who helped provide supplies for the American and French armies during the Revolutionary War.

Who is Tom Brokaw?
A US journalist of Dutch descent who was anchorman for the *NBC Nightly News with Tom Brokaw*.

Who was Walter Cronkite?
A US journalist and anchorman for CBS News who was of Dutch descent.

Who is Ray Noorda?
The son of Dutch immigrants and the only person who has earned the right to be called the Father of Network Computing. He launched the Utah Information Technology Sector, the fastest growing industry in Utah during the past few decades.

Who was Cornelius Vanderbilt II?
A US inventor of Dutch descent who registered over 30 patents including a corrugated firebox for locomotives which greatly improved efficiency, a cylindrical tank car for transporting bulk oil and other liquids, and a revolutionary type of locomotive tender.

Who was Lee De Forest?
The inventor of the Audion vacuum tube used for radio transmissions. He was a direct descendant of Jessé de Forest, the leader of a group of

Walloon Huguenots who fled Europe in the seventeenth century due to religious persecution.

Who was Thomas Edison?
Although he did not invent the light bulb, he made it commercially viable by inventing power distribution for electric lighting. His ancestors were Dutch.

Who was Peter Zondervan?
The Dutch-American who was the major co-founder of Zondervan Corporation of Grand Rapids, Michigan, one of the nation's largest publishers of religious books, including bibles.

Who was Martin van Buren?
US President from 1837 to 1841 and of Dutch ancestry.

Who was Eleanor Roosevelt?
Wife of US President Franklin Delano Roosevelt and a well-known humanitarian who fought for equal rights for women and African Americans. Her ancestors were Dutch.

Who was Oliver Wendell Holmes, Jr?
Of Dutch descent, he was appointed to the US Supreme Court in 1902 and was one of the most widely cited US Supreme Court justices in history. He served until age 90.

Sports and Games

Sports

Of the 16 million people in the Netherlands, over 5 million are registered members of sports clubs. The country has thousands of organizations ranging from national sports authorities down to local clubs catering to all ages.

Football, which Americans call soccer, is the number-one sport for both playing and watching. The big three football clubs are: Ajax Amsterdam, Rotterdam Feyenoord, and PSV Eindhoven.

Ice skating is also an important part of the Dutch sports heritage. Once hugely popular, it has recently been relegated from frozen waterways to indoor ice rinks. Speed skating, not figure skating, is a national obsession. The province of Friesland is the skating heartland and hosts the longest skating marathon on natural ice in the world, the Eleven Cities race.

Other popular sports include hockey, cycling, tennis, equestrian sports, badminton, and squash. Baseball and softball are becoming popular.

Indoor sports include gymnastics, indoor football, volleyball, basketball, and handball. Sailing, boxing, table tennis, and swimming are minority sports.

Sports Trivia

True or false: Cycling is a popular sport in the Netherlands.
True. In fact, there are more bicycles than people in the country.

Can you ride a bike across the entire country?
Yes. Three international cycling routes cross the Netherlands, among which the North Sea Route along the Dutch coastline is especially attractive.

What sports are available on Dutch beaches?
Swimming, jet skiing, and water skiing.

Where is the best place for wind surfing and kite surfing?
The north beach on the island of Terschelling.

How do the Dutch use their many miles of canals?
The numerous interconnected canals and waterways that cross the country are perfect for canoeing, kayaking, and rafting.

True or false: The Netherlands is considered the best country in the world for in-line skating.
True. Skaters use the country's many approved bike lanes.

Are there public golf courses?
Yes, as well as many golf courses connected to hotels.

What outdoor sports areas are popular in warm weather?
Outdoor swimming pools, aqua parks, and tennis courts.

What is the most popular walking area?
The two national parks in the Veluwe ridge hills. Veluwezoom and De Hoge Veluwe each have walking trails.

True or false: All roadways in the Netherlands are designed with bike lanes.
True. In fact, in some cities cars are banned and bikes are the only transportation.

Game

Sjoelbak is a shuffleboard game, and one of the most beloved games in the Netherlands. It is similar to English shuffleboard which began in the sixteenth century when players shuffled metal weights on a table. The following is modified for residents.

Number of players. Six.

Materials. An 8' long by 25" wide wooden board and four 6" high by 6" wide arches attached to the board. Thirty wooden disks, each three inches wide and one inch thick.

Alternative board and materials. A 24" by 36" sheet of white poster board, four different colored sponges, glue, and 30 plastic bottle caps. Cut half circles into the dry sponges so they look like arches and glue them in a row across the 24" end of the poster board. Let dry so the sponges are attached firmly to the board. Place this board on a table and let residents aim the bottle caps at the sponges.

To play. Place the shuffleboard on a long table and allow the residents to take turns with the goal of sliding as many of the 30 wooden disks through the four small colored arches. Each color is worth a different point: 1 for green, 2 for red, 3 for yellow, and 4 for blue. Each player has three chances to slide pucks into the scoring boxes.

Winner. The player with the highest number of points wins the game.

ICHI benefits. Mental functions of language, speech, articulation and joint mobility, muscle force, and control of voluntary movement.

Music and Dance

Music

Dutch folk music was originally preserved by the oral tradition, one generation teaching the songs to the next. The oldest recorded Dutch songbook, the *Antwerps Liedboek*, originated in 1544 and was the first in a series of songbook releases in the Netherlands.

The term Levenslied was first used by Jean-Louis Pisuisse in 1908 to describe a much loved form of Dutch music. Levenslied are simple ballads, typically with a poignant theme such as unrequited love. The invention of the gramophone allowed Dutch musicians to attract a wider audience. At the end of World War II, because Dutch youth were listening to music coming from the UK and the US, enthusiasm for the Levenslied waned.

The influence of pop music resulted in several Dutch singers, including Eddy Christiani and Willy Alberti, having some success in the US. During the seventies pop and rock bands began to steer away from the Dutch language which was particularly associated with the out-of-style Levenslied. As increasing numbers of Dutch musicians sang in English, their chance of outside fame grew. Shocking Blue made it to the top of the foreign charts with *Venus* and Golden Earring had an international hit with *Radar Love*.

The English language trend was bucked somewhat in the northern province of Fryslan, where a handful of folk groups continued. The trend for singing in English began to reverse throughout the country during the eighties. In the 1990s many famous pop stars and successful bands routinely sang in Dutch. The Levenslied returned to the Dutch music scene in the late 1980s and remains popular.

Music Videos

Baroque Music from the Netherlands: Accessed April 3, 2015,
  https://www.youtube.com/watch?v=i-x3g0OIaJ0
Holland and his [its] music: Accessed April 3, 2015,
  https://www.youtube.com/watch?v=QJwWZh3aEoM
Netherlands Music and Images: Accessed April 3, 2015,
  https://www.youtube.com/watch?v=GP2OxBrdHTE
Stilte voor de storm by Dutch folk group Pekel: Accessed April 3, 2015.
  https://www.youtube.com/watch?v=Hr7r63I-Jf4
Traditional Dutch Folk Music: Accessed April 3, 2015,
  PLlYNbPbxv7owWy6zQBkQ0hS5AjeOArnAD

Dance

Dutch folk dance has been associated with clogging, although in practice clogs limit dance moves. Thus Dutch folk dance is mostly danced in shoes, also because historically the Dutch danced in shoes worn as part of their church-going clothing. Traditionally clogs were used only for work.

Most folk dances regarded as Dutch are actually of Scots origin, such as *Skotse trije*, *Skotse fjouwer*, and *Horlepiep of hakke toone*. In the Eastern Netherlands dances such as *Driekusman*, *Hoksebarger*, *Veleta*, *Kruispolka*, and the *Spaanse Wals* are of German origin.

Dance Videos

Dutch Clog Dance with Wooden Shoes: Accessed April 3, 2015,
    https://www.youtube.com/watch?v=811WRua-Yzk
Dutch Folk Dance: Accessed April 3, 2015,
    https://www.youtube.com/watch?v=woo2dgkqGl4
Dutch Folk Dance 2: Accessed April 3, 2015,
    https://www.youtube.com/watch?v=8e_sz-JCGV0
Dutch Folk Dance at Amsterdam: Accessed April 3, 2015,
    https://vimeo.com/11986061
Tulip Time: Accessed April 3, 2015, http://www.tuliptime.com/dutch-heritage/dutch-dance/

Music and Dance Trivia

Who was Jan Pieterszoon Sweelinck?
A Dutch composer, organist, and pedagogue whose work straddled the end of the Renaissance and beginning of the Baroque eras. Sweelinck was a master improviser and was known as the Orpheus of Amsterdam.

Who was Jacob van Eyck?
A blind recorder and organ virtuoso who composed a unique collection of flute music.

Who was Alphons Diepenbrock?
A sixteenth-century composer.

Do Dutch dancers dance to the melody or the bass line?
The bass line of the music.

True or false: Dutch clogs are made entirely of wood.
True.

True or false: Most Dutch folk dances are designed to be performed by a single dancer.
False: Dutch dances are mainly group dances.

Who is Misha Mengelberg?
A Dutch jazz pianist and composer.

Who was Willem Breuker?
A jazz bandleader, composer, arranger, saxophonist, and bass clarinetist.

What band won the Eurovision Song Contest of 1975 with the song *Ding-A-Dong*?
Teach-In.

What is the name for Dutch electronic music?
Gabber.

Food

Dutch foods come from a mixture of cultures. Breakfast and lunch are simple meals of bread, fruit, and dairy products. Supper is usually a warm meal served between 6 and 7 pm. Most restaurants close between 9 and 10 pm.

Some Dutch meals to consider sampling are *snert* which is a pea soup with sausages and *stamppot*, a popular winter stew of vegetables, potatoes, and meat.

For something sweet, try *poffertjes*, a kind of mini-pancake but thicker and sweeter and often served with sugar and butter. The most popular snack is *patatje met*, French fries dipped in mayonnaise.

For a late afternoon snack, try *bitterballen*, small fried balls of beef ragout. Another sweet is *muisjes*, an aniseed comfit eaten as a bread topping and available with a pink, blue, or white outer layer of sugar.

The country's most famous dessert is *stroopwafel*, a waffle cookie made from baked batter and sliced horizontally. The two thin layers are then filled with a special sweet and sticky syrup. The stiff batter for the waffles is made from butter, flour, yeast, milk, brown sugar, and eggs. Stroopwafel are served with a cup of coffee or tea.

The *stroopwafel* originated in Gouda, a place south of Amsterdam, during the late eighteenth or early nineteenth century, created by a baker using leftover breadcrumbs sweetened with syrup.

Recipe

Dutch Cookies.
Ingredients.
¾ cup butter
¾ cup sugar
1⅓ cups flour
Pinch of salt
1 tablespoon cinnamon.
½ cup finely chopped walnuts
Preparation. For topping, combine ¼ cup of sugar and the walnuts, and set aside. Cream together butter, ½ cup of sugar, flour, salt, and cinnamon until the mixture looks like cornmeal. Pat the dough into a foil-lined baking sheet. Sprinkle topping over the dough. Bake at 350 degrees F. for 20 minutes. Cut into bars. Serves 20.

Food Trivia

True or false: Seventy percent of the world's bacon comes from the Netherlands.
True.

True or false: Gin was invented in the Netherlands.
True. Invented in the sixteenth century, it was called *jenever* and was originally for medical use.

What is the national dish of the Netherlands?
Herring with chopped raw onions.

How much of the national dish does the average citizen eat?
About five full fish per year.

How much beer does the average person drink?
74 liters per year.

How much coffee do the Dutch drink per day?
3.2 cups per person.

How many kinds of licorice sweets are sold?
80 varieties.

What Dutch brewery exports to over 70 countries?
Heineken.

How much beer does Heineken export?
50 percent of its production.

When did the Dutch begin making cheese?
400 AD.

Customs

Weddings

The bridal shower tradition originated in Holland. According to legend, if a Dutch bride's father disapproved of her choice of a husband he would not offer her a dowry. When this occurred, the bride's friends would shower her with gifts of household items usually included in the dowry.

If the family approved of the groom, the bride would receive a trousseau from her parents and her future father-in-law would give her a *chatelaine*, a chain or rope made of silver or leather that held various items such as a pair of scissors, a pincushion, a needle case, a small knife, and a mirror.

Traditionally, before the wedding ceremony bridesmaids filled the bride's basket with green garlands and flowers and decorated the groom's pipe with garlands and ribbons. The bride's house was painted green and the families hosted a party where the couple would sit on a throne beneath pine trees as their guests came to bless them and wish them happiness.

During the ceremony the bride and groom walked on a bed of flowers to the altar and flowers were tossed at them as they departed. During the reception traditional items were served, including sweetmeats called bridal sugar, and spiced wine which was known as bride's tears.

Instead of tossing her bouquet, the bride would toss her crown. Whoever caught it would be the next to be married.

Children

Thirty percent of all births in the Netherlands are home births. Mothers-to-be are encouraged to attend prenatal yoga classes to help with the process of labor and delivery. About ten percent of women receive pain medication during labor. In the US the Centers for Disease Control report that about 60 percent of women in labor receive pain medication.

Prior to the home birth, insurance companies send to the home a *kraampakket* which contains the materials needed for a home birth. Most births are attended by a midwife and a maternity care assistant. If the child in born in a hospital, the mother and child are sent home a few hours after the birth.

After either a home or hospital birth the maternity care assistant visits the home within hours to provide *kraamzorg*, including care for the new mother and infant, light household duties, guidance on breast feeding and baby care, and looking after other family members, such as other children, for about a week.

Within three days of birth, every child born in the Netherlands must be registered at the municipal population affairs office and receives a birth certificate. Registration information includes given name or names, surname, sex, place of birth, date and time of birth, given name(s) and surname of each parent, and place and date of birth of each parent.

In the Netherlands if a man and a woman are married or are in a registered partnership and have a child, the mother's husband is automatically designated the child's lawful father, whether or not he is the child's biological father. If they are not married, a father may choose if he wants his name added to the birth certificate.

Holidays

January 1. New Year's Day
Variable date. Easter
Variable date. Easter Monday
April 27. King's Birthday

Variable date. Whit Monday, the day after Pentecost
December 26. Second Day of Christmas

Customs Trivia

Why do newlyweds plant lilies of the valley around their house?
To symbolize the return of happiness with each season, renewing their love.

What is a Dutch wish tree?
At the wedding reception a beautiful tree branch is placed next to the bride and groom's table with paper leaves attached so guests can write a special wish for the happy couple on the leaves.

What do the Dutch eat to celebrate the birth of a baby?
Rusk with aniseed comfit.

True or false: Guests dine with the bride before the wedding.
True. Before the wedding day, guests visit the bride's house where they eat *bruid suikas*, a traditional sweetmeat served with spiced wine.

True or false: Guests are invited to a party prior to the wedding ceremony.
True. Many Dutch couples invite guests to a short party before the wedding and offer drinks, nuts, olive, and other tasty finger food before proceeding to the wedding venue.

True or false: Gifts are unwrapped at the wedding reception.
True. Traditionally gifts are unwrapped immediately and passed around to be admired and the giver thanked.

What is a must at every wedding reception?
A large silver bowl filled with brandy and raisins that is passed around as the song *How sweet it is where friendship dwells…* is sung.

What is a traditional marriage proposal?
When a boy wanted to ask a girl for marriage, he would hand-carve a pair of clogs with beautiful designs. He would then place them secretly at the girl's doorstep during the night. The boy would go back to the girl's house the next morning and if the girl was wearing the clogs, that showed she had accepted his marriage proposal.

Why do brides and grooms wear wooden shoes on the wedding day?
For tradition and good luck.

What happens to the wooden shoes after the wedding?
They are hung on the wall of the newlyweds' home.

More Resources

DVDs

Back Roads of Europe Southern Limburg The Netherlands, DVD, Travel Video Store, 2007.
Back Roads of Europe Southwest of Drenthe The Netherlands, DVD, Travel Video Store, 2007.
Back Roads of Europe The Delfland Route The Netherlands, DVD, Travel Video Store, 2007.
Back Roads of Europe Western Zeeland Flanders The Netherlands, DVD, Travel Video Store, 2007.
Back Roads of Europe Westerwolde The Netherlands, DVD, Travel Video Store, 2007.

Books

DK Eyewitness Travel Guide: The Netherlands (DK Publishing, 2014).
Steves, R. *Pocket Amsterdam* (Avalon Travel Publishing, 2014).
Steves, R. Rick Steves' *Amsterdam & the Netherlands* (Avalon Travel Publishing, 2015).
Ver Berkmoes, R. and Zimmerman, K. *Lonely Planet The Netherlands*. (Lonely Planet, 2013).
Zimmerman, K. and LeNevez, C. *Lonely Planet Amsterdam* (Lonely Planet, 2014).

Websites

Government of the Netherlands: Accessed April 4, 2015,
http://www.government.nl/
Holland: Accessed April 4, 2015,
http://www.holland.com/global/tourism.htm urism.htm

Map of Netherlands: Accessed April 4, 2015,
   http://www.worldatlas.com/webimage/countrys/europe/nl.htm
US Relations With the Netherlands: Accessed April 4, 2015,
   http://www.state.gov/r/pa/ei/bgn/3204.htm

Photos

Netherlands: Accessed April 4, 2015, http://www.lonelyplanet.com/the-
   netherlands/images
Netherlands: Accessed April 4, 2015, .
   http://travel.nationalgeographic.com/travel/countries/netherlands-
   guide/
Netherland Photos: Accessed April 4, 2015,
   http://www.trekearth.com/gallery/Europe/Netherlands/
Pictures of the Netherlands: Accessed. April 4, 2015,
   http://www.globetrotter.photography/holland/holland.html
The Netherlands: Accessed April 4, 2015,
   http://www.tripadvisor.com/LocationPhotos-g188553-
   The_Netherlands.html

References

60 Interesting Facts about the Netherlands: Accessed April 2, 2015,
   http://www.weekendnotes.com/interesting-facts-about-netherlands/
Country of Netherlands Coloring Pages: Accessed April 3, 2015,
   http://www.coloring.ws/netherlands.htm
Dutch-Americans: Accessed April 3, 2015,
   http://www.newnetherlandinstitute.org/history-and-
   heritage/dutch_americans/accomplishments
Dutch Folk Dance: Accessed April 3, 2015,
   http://www.ask.com/wiki/Dutch_folk_dance?o=2800&qsrc=999&ad=doubleDown
   &an=apn&ap=ask.com
Dutch Wedding Reception Traditions: Accessed April 3, 2015,
   http://www.toptableplanner.com/blog/dutch-wedding-reception-traditions
Dutch Wedding Traditions and Customs: Accessed April 3, 2015, http://www.beau-
   coup.com/dutch-wedding-traditions.htm
Easy Dutch Cookies: Accessed April 3, 2015,
   http://www.cooks.com/rec/doc/prt/0,1718,148184-255206,00.html
Family Law: Accessed April 4, 2015, http://www.government.nl/issues/family-law/birth-
   of-a-child

Holland. Dutch Cuisine: Accessed April 3, 2015,
   http://www.holland.com/us/tourism/article/dutch-cuisine.htm
Maternity Matters: What to Expect in the Netherlands: Accessed April 4, 2015,
   http://www.expatica.com/nl/healthcare/Maternity-matters-What-to-expect-in-the-
   Netherlands_101827.html
Music from the Netherlands. Accessed April 3, 2015,
   http://dutchcommunity.com/2012/05/30/music-from-the-netherlands/
Music of the Netherlands: Accessed April 3, 2015,
   http://www.worldmusic.net/guide/music-of-the-netherlands/
Netherlands: Accessed April 3, 2015, http://www.booking.com/hotel/nl/b-amp-b-
   helmers.en-us.html?aid=318615;label=New_English_EN_CAUS_5226331825-
   t3Fsf96*29kPJ0Wd8uRMegS46623191905%3Apl%3Ata%3Ap1%3Ap2%3Aac%3
   Aap1t2%3Anes;sid=67d1273fe34830b3a4b800c7076086b4;dcid=4;src=clp;opened
   LpRecProp=1;ccpi=1
Netherlands History: Accessed April 3, 2015,
   http://www.amsterdam.info/netherlands/history/
Sport in Netherland: Accessed April 3, 2015, http://www.europe-
   cities.com/en/672/netherlands/sport/
Sports in Netherlands: Accessed April 3, 2015, http://www.nlplanet.com/nlguides/dutch-
   sport
The Netherlands: Accessed April 3, 2015,
   http://www.infoplease.com/country/netherlands.html
The Netherlands: Accessed April 3, 2015,
   http://www.travelmath.com/from/Seattle,+WA/to/Amsterdam,+Netherlands
Traditional Dutch Games for Children: Accessed April 3, 2015,
   http://expatsincebirth.com/2013/04/29/traditional-dutch-games-for-children-
   sjoelbak-koekhappen-en-spijkerpoep/
Viator Insider's Guide to Amsterdam: Accessed April 3, 2015,
   http://www.viator.com/Amsterdam/d525/top-attractions#attractions

NORTHERN IRELAND

Basics

Geography

Northern Ireland is composed of 26 districts derived from the boroughs of Belfast and Londonderry and the counties of Antrim, Armagh, Down, Fermanagh, Londonderry, and Tyrone. These are commonly called Ulster, though the territory does not include the entire ancient province of Ulster. The country is slightly larger than Connecticut.

Language

The common languages are English, Irish, and Ulster Scots.

History

Ulster was part of Ireland until the mid-1500s when England under Queen Elizabeth I triumphed over three Irish rebellions and confiscated the lands, settling the Scots Presbyterians in Ulster. In 1641–1651 another rebellion was brutally crushed by Oliver Cromwell, resulting in the settlement of Anglican Englishmen in Ulster. Subsequent political policy favoring Protestants over Catholics encouraged further Protestant settlement in Northern Ireland.

Northern Ireland did not separate from the South until 1886, when William Gladstone presented his proposal for Irish home rule. The Protestants in the North feared domination by the Catholic majority. Northern Ireland became a separate country in 1922 with a semiautonomous parliament in Belfast and a Crown-appointed governor advised by a cabinet composed of the prime minister and eight ministers. It also had 12 representatives in the House of Commons in London.

The Irish Republican Army (IRA) sought to end the partition of Ireland. In 1966–1969, rioting and street fighting between Protestants and Catholics in Londonderry were caused both by extremist nationalist Protestants who feared that Catholics might attain a local majority and by Catholics demonstrating for civil rights.

Fighting, bombings, and conflicts known as "the Troubles" continued through the 1970s, 1980s, and 1990s until the Good Friday Agreement of April 10, 1998. This required Protestants to share political power with the Catholic minority and gave the Republic of Ireland a voice in Northern Irish affairs. In turn, Irish Catholics agreed to suspend their goal of a united Ireland unless and until the day when the largely Protestant North voted in favor of such an arrangement.

Map and Flag

Create a flag: Accessed March 7, 2015,
    http://www.activityvillage.co.uk/northern-ireland-flag-printables
Create a map: Accessed March 7, 2015,-
    http://www.enchantedlearning.com/europe/ireland/activity.shtml

Travel

Distance

From New York, NY, to Belfast, Northern Ireland is 3,181 miles. Flight time is 6 hours 52 minutes.

From Chicago, IL, to Belfast, Northern Ireland is 3,650 miles. Flight time is 7 hours 48 minutes.

From Dallas, TX, to Belfast, Northern Ireland is 4,452 miles. Flight time is 9 hours 24 minutes.

From Seattle, WA, to Belfast Northern Ireland is 4,481 miles. Flight time is 9 hours 28 minutes.

Hotels

Ballyrobin Country Lodge. Located on Ballyrobin Road in Belfast near Clotworthy Arts Centre and Antrim Castle, it features 24-hour coffee service.

City Hotel. Located on Queens Quay in Londonderry, it features a hot tub, steam room, and an indoor heated swimming pool.

La Mon Hotel and Country Club. Located on Gransha Road in Belfast, it features an outdoor pool, a children's pool, a tennis court, and two gyms. Guests can enjoy a complimentary Irish breakfast each morning and dine at the two onsite restaurants.

Maldron Hotel Derry. Located on Butcher Street in Londonderry, it features the Stir Restaurant which offers a full Ulster or continental breakfast and the Lyric Bar which offers complimentary live entertainment during the weekend.

Somerton House Bed and Breakfast. Located on Lansdowne Road in Belfast, it features in-room coffee makers and is within one mile of Fortwilliam Golf Club, Belfast Castle, St. Anne's Cathedral, and Belfast City Hall.

Landmarks

Giant's Causeway. Thousands of interlocking basalt columns in a headland facing the North Atlantic Ocean's North Channel towards Scotland. Geologists believe that these natural formations were the result of intense volcanic eruptions in the area around 50 to 60 million years ago. It was declared a World Heritage Site by the UNESCO in 1986 and a National Nature Reserve by Northern Ireland in 1987.

Londonderry. Also known as Derry. The best-preserved walled town on the island of Ireland, it is one of the finest examples of a walled city in Europe. Completed in 1618, the walls are up to 26 feet high and 35 feet thick in spots and feature watchtowers and cannons.

St. Patrick's Trail. A 92-mile drive that includes 15 sites connected to the life of St. Patrick, including sites in Bangor, the Ards Peninsula, Downpatrick, Newry, and Armagh. St. Patrick Center is located between the Mountains of Mourne and scenic Strangford Lough and is dedicated to the history of the saint and reconciliation between Ireland and Northern Ireland.

Saul Church. Located two miles outside Downpatrick, it was built in 1932, to commemorate Saint Patrick's first church in Ireland.

Tower Museum. Located in Londonderry, it features an exhibit about La Trinidad Valencera, one of the largest ships in the Armada Fleet, which foundered in Kinnagoe Bay in County Donegal during a violent storm in 1588. It was discovered nearly 400 years later by divers from the City of Derry Sub Aqua Club.

Travel Trivia

What is the capital of Northern Ireland?
Belfast.

What is the Northern Ireland flag?
The Union Flag, which is the official flag of the United Kingdom of Great Britain and Northern Ireland, is the only flag used by the government in Northern Ireland.

What is the official name of Northern Ireland?
The United Kingdom of Great Britain and Northern Ireland.

What famous ship was built in Belfast?
HMS Titanic.

What is the longest river in Northern Ireland?
The River Bann, at 80 miles.

What is the largest lake?
The Lough Neagh is 151 miles and is the largest freshwater lake in the British Isles.

What is the national anthem?
Danny Boy.

What famous breweries are located in Northern Ireland?
Guinness, Smithwicks, and Harp Lager.

What is the highest point in the country?
Slieve Donard Mountain at 2,782 feet.

What is the legend of Giant's Causeway?
Legend says mythical warrior Finn McCool built it to cross the sea to do battle against a much bigger Scottish archrival, Benandonner. Finn's wife

disguised her husband as their baby son. Seeing an infant so huge, Benandonner concluded that Finn, the father, must be a giant. The Scottish warrior fled but destroyed Finn's bridge which then became the natural wonder located in Antrim, Northern Ireland.

What does the sign "You are now entering Free Derry" mean?
The fighting between Catholics wanting a united Ireland and Protestants wanting Northern Ireland to be part of the United Kingdom is believed to have started in Derry in the 1960s. The sign in Bogside, a Catholic neighborhood, proclaims the political differences.

Who was C. S. Lewis?
Clive Staples Lewis was born in 1898 and became a writer. He was a Fellow and Tutor in English Literature at Oxford University until 1954, when he was unanimously elected to the Chair of Medieval and Renaissance Literature at Cambridge University, a position he held until his retirement. He wrote more than 30 books including *Mere Christianity* and *The Chronicles of Narnia*.

Who was William Burke?
A serial killer born in Northern Ireland who committed 16 murders in Edinburgh, Scotland, over 10 months in 1828. He sold the victims' bodies to Doctor Robert Knox to be used for dissection.

How many counties make-up Northern Ireland?
Six.

What are the major cities in Northern Ireland?
Belfast, Londonderry, Lisburn, Newtonabbey, Bangor, and Craigavon.

What is the ruling body of Northern Ireland called?
The Northern Ireland Assembly.

Who was Sir James Martin?
The inventor of the airplane ejector seat.

Who was Harry Ferguson?
The inventor of the modern agricultural tractor.

Who was Frank Pantridge?
The inventor of the portable defibrillator.

Who was Sir Henry Pottinger?
A soldier and governor of Hong Kong when the area was under British control.

America's Roots

Who was Bill Clinton?
The US president whose Blythe and Ayer ancestors were among 250,000 immigrants from the north of Ireland who settled along the American frontier prior to 1800.

Who was James Buchanan?
The US president who said, "My Ulster blood is a priceless heritage." His family were originally from Deroran, near Omagh in County Tyrone.

Who was Ulysses Simpson Grant?
The US president whose maternal great-grandfather John Simpson was born at Dergenagh, County Tyrone. Grant visited his ancestral homeland in 1878.

Who was William Barclay "Bat" Masterson?
A US gunfighter, buffalo hunter, frontier lawman, and newspaperman. He was the son of Catherine McGurk who was from Northern Ireland.

Who was Stephen Foster?
Born in America, he was a songwriter and the great-grandson of Alexander Foster of Derry, Ireland.

Who was Matthew Thornton?
A signer of the Declaration of Independence who was born in Ireland.

Who was George Taylor?
A signer the Declaration of Independence who was born in Ireland.

Who was Richard Milhous Nixon?
The thirty-seventh President of the United States. His ancestor Isaac Brown was born in Ireland in 1771, and both his ancestors named James Moore were born in Ballymoney, County Antrim, Ireland in 1777 and 1759. Another of his ancestors, Thomas Milhous, was born in Carrickfergus, County Antrim, Ireland, in 1699.

Who was Ronald Wilson Reagan?
The fortieth US President. His great-grandfather Michael Reagan was believed to be from Ireland, possibly baptized there in 1829 in Ballyporeen, and immigrated to the US via Canada in 1858.

Who was Andrew Jackson?
The seventh US President. His parents Andrew Jackson and Elizabeth Hutchinson were from Carrickfergus, County Antrim, Ireland, as was his paternal grandfather, Hugh Jackson.

Who is Michael Fassbender?
An actor and Oscar-nominated star of *12 Years a Slave*, *X-Men: Origins*, and *Inglourious Basterds*. His mother hails from County Antrim in Northern Ireland.

Who was Arthur Guinness?
He was born in Ireland and founded the Guinness brewery. He fathered 21 children.

Who was John Dunlap?
The first printer of the US Declaration of Independence, he was from Northern Ireland.

Who is Denis Leary?
A comedian and the son of Nora Sullivan and John Leary, both Irish immigrants.

Who is Regis Philbin?
A well-known TV personality who co-hosted his own daytime talk show for almost three decades and has Irish ancestors.

Sports and Games

Sports

Most sports, including rugby union, gaelic games, basketball, rugby league, hockey, and cricket, are organized on an all-Ireland basis. Some others, such as association football (which Americans call soccer) and netball are organized on a separate basis for Northern Ireland.

The Irish Football Association (IFA) is the organizing body for football (soccer) in Northern Ireland. The Northern Ireland Women's Football Association (NIWFA) sponsors a Women's Cup, Women's League, and the Northern Ireland women's national football team.

Many football fans in Northern Ireland prefer to support teams from England such as Manchester United and Liverpool and teams from Scotland such as Celtics and Rangers.

Netball is a ball sport played by two teams of seven players. Its development, derived from early versions of basketball, began in England in the 1890s. By 1960, international playing rules had been standardized for the game and the International Federation of Netball and Women's Basketball.

Games are played on a rectangular court with raised goal rings at each end. Each team attempts to score goals by passing a ball down the court and shooting it through its goal ring. Players are assigned specific positions which define their roles within the team and restrict their movement to certain areas of the court. During general play, a player with the ball can hold on to it for only three seconds before shooting for a goal or passing to another player. The winning team is the one that scores the most goals. Netball games are 60 minutes long.

Other sports enjoyed in Northern Ireland include Gaelic football, hurling, cricket, golf, and Gaelic handball.

Sports Trivia

Who was George Best?
A football (soccer) player born in Belfast who was the European Footballer of the year in 1968.

Who is Norman Whiteside?
A football (soccer) player born in Belfast who is the youngest player to ever take part in the World Cup.

Who is Darren Clarke?
A golfer born in Dungannon who has won 22 worldwide tournaments.

Who was Dave McCauley?
A boxer born in Belfast who won the International Boxing Federation (IBF) World Title in the Flyweight category.

Who is Alex Higgins?
A snooker player credited with bringing the game to Northern Ireland.

What is snooker?
A game using a cue and 22 balls on a table covered by a green cloth with a pocket in each of the four corners.

How big is a snooker table?
12 feet by 6 feet.

What is potting?
A snooker term for getting a ball into the pocket.

Where was snooker invented?
Legend says it was invented by British army officers in Jabalpur, India.

Who is Eddie Irvine?
A retired Formula One racer from Northern Ireland who was runner-up in the 1999 Formula One World Drivers' Championship.

Game

Rings. A toss game played indoors, often in a pub, and requiring a wall board with hooks, each worth a different value. Players stand behind a line and toss stiff rope rings at the hooks with the goal of scoring points each time they place a ring on a hook. The game uses a cross-piece base with four corner posts and a center post. Each post is worth a different number of points. Players toss stiff rope rings, called quoits, at the posts to score points each time a ring lands over a post.

Number of players. Five, or two teams with five players on each team.

Materials. Modified for residents: One over-the-door coat rack with five or six hooks. For residents in wheelchairs, hook this rack to the side of a coffee cart as that will place the hooks directly across from the arms of the players. Paint the hooks, red, yellow, blue, green, black, and white. Make 20 stiff rope rings by cutting rope into 8" lengths and tying each length into a circle. Stiffen the rope circles by letting them sit overnight in starch, then removing them and letting them dry.

To play. Five players sit about three feet from a coat rack. Give each player four rings. Have them take turns one at a time throwing the rings.

Give each hook a color. Each red is one point, blue two points, yellow three points, green four points, black five points, and white six points.

Winner. The player with the most points after all the rings are tossed.

ICHI benefits. Mental functions of language, speech, articulation and voluntary control of movement, muscle force, and mobility of joints.

Music and Dance

Music

Irish music incorporates fiddles, bagpipes, drums, flutes, and harps. Folk music is performed in pubs and parades. The Ulster National Orchestra in Belfast and the Philharmonic Society are the leading classical musical groups. In the past decade, traditional Irish music has grown very popular outside the country.

Northern Ireland has also produced rock stars such as Van Morrison and bands including *Stiff Little Fingers*, who first formed in 1977 and are still touring and recording today, as well as *The Outcasts* and *Rudi*.

Punk rock stars from Derry include *The Undertones*, the post-punk/New Wave band that brought us the song *Teenage Kicks*.

Since 2000 the bands *Ash* and *Snow Patrol* have achieved worldwide success, each selling millions of albums.

Music Videos

A Song for Northern Ireland Peace: Accessed March 7, 2015,
    https://www.youtube.com/watch?v=owC9lW_xE28
Meet Silhouette: Accessed March 7, 2015,
    https://www.youtube.com/watch?v=PZvi1HCt_SI
Northern Ireland Music Highlights: Accessed April 5, 2015,
    https://www.youtube.com/watch?v=2A6K27OALH4
Northern Ireland Music Highlights during Belfast Music Week: Accessed
    March 7, 2015, https://www.youtube.com/watch?v=2A6K27OALH4
Northern Ireland Song: Accessed April 5, 2015,
    https://www.youtube.com/watch?v=6tQB9gSOKOo

Dance

Historians believe that Irish dancing began with the ancient Druids who danced in religious rituals honoring the sun. These ancient practices could be the beginnings of the popular ring dances performed today. When the Celts arrived in Ireland over 2,000 years ago, they brought their European folk dances.

The Anglo-Norman conquest of Ireland in the twelfth century brought Norman dances including the *Carol*, a popular Norman dance in which the leader sang and was surrounded by a circle of dancers who replied with the same song.

Three principal Irish dances are often mentioned in sixteenth-century writing: the *Irish Hey*, the *Rinnce Fada* (long dance), and the *Trenchmore*. In a letter written to Queen Elizabeth I in 1569, Sir Henry Sydney said of girls performing an Irish jig, "They are very beautiful, magnificently dressed, and first class dancers."

During the mid-sixteenth century the *Hey* was a popular dance in which female dancers wound around their partners in a forerunner of the present day reel.

Irish dancing was accompanied by music played on the bagpipes and the harp. Dancing was also performed during wakes. The mourners danced to bagpipe music in a ring around the coffin.

Solo dancing or step dancing began at the end of the eighteenth century.

The costumes worn by Irish dancers today are based on the Irish peasant dress worn 200 years ago. Most of the dresses are adorned with hand-embroidered Celtic designs. Men wear a plain kilt and jacket with a folded cloak draped from the shoulder. Male and female dancers wear hornpipe shoes for step dancing and soft shoes similar to ballet pumps for reels and jigs.

Dance Videos

Hoop and Fire Dancer: Accessed March 7, 2015,
    https://search.yahoo.com/search?ei=utf-8&fr=ytff1-
    yff27&p=northern%20ireland%20dancers&type=
Northern Ireland Championships 2014: Accessed April 5, 2015,
    https://www.youtube.com/watch?v=2rkmNRRI74I

Northern Ireland Dancers Lisbum: Accessed March 7, 2015,
    https://www.youtube.com/watch?v=IG5V9dIU0n0
Wilbur in Northern Ireland: How to Irish Dance: Accessed April 5, 2015,
    https://www.youtube.com/watch?v=EVlfKl9NrGY

Music and Dance Trivia

Who is Ruth Augilera?
A professional singer from Belfast who played the leading role of Mimi
in *Rent* in London's West End.

Who was Gary Moore?
A guitarist for the band Thin Lizzy who died in 2011.

Who is Vivian Campbell?
A guitarist for the band Def Leppard.

Where did the band The Answer get its start?
County Down in Northern Ireland in 2000.

What was Van Morrison's big hit song in 1967?
Brown Eyed Girl.

Who is Feargal Sharkey?
A punk rock singer who recorded *Never Never* and *A Good Heart.*

What is Celtic Storm?
A professional dance company from Northern Ireland.

Who is Tristan MacManus?
An Irish dancer who appeared on the TV show *Dancing with the Stars.*

Where can you attend a ballet in Northern Ireland?
The Opera House in Belfast.

What is *Let the Dance Begin*?
A sculpture of dancers, in Strabane, Northern Ireland.

Food

Northern Ireland's culinary heritage reflects the mixing of the Ulster-
Scots with Irish heritage and traditions. Traditionally the Ulster Fry was

eaten for breakfast every day, but nowadays that pleasure is saved for the weekend plus indulging in a *sausage soda* (soda bread filled with sausage, bacon, and egg) or a *bacon bap* (bacon sandwich on buttered bread) on a weekday.

Another Northern Ireland breakfast treat is porridge made with rolled oats, milk or water, and a pinch of salt. Some add cream rather than milk, brown sugar, and occasionally a dash of Bushmills whiskey. A common mid-morning snack is a cup of tea or a very milky coffee, often accompanied by a scone, fruit cake, sticky sweet tray bake, or cream cake.

A favorite for the main meal of the day is Irish stew, a casserole traditionally made with lamb, potatoes, carrots, and onions. However, the Ulster variety is made with steak pieces cooked to a peppery slush and often served with thick slices of buttered bread.

Other meats and sides for the main meal are steak and Guinness pies, Ardglass potted herring, butcher's sausages, pasties, and *boxty*.

Recipe

Ulster Fry. Once a traditional breakfast, it is now served mostly on weekends and holidays.

Ingredients.

2 eggs
2 slices of bacon
2 sausages
Olive oil
2 slices potato bread
Sliced tomatoes and a frying pan.

Preparation. Add a drizzle of olive oil to a frying pan and heat over a low and slow heat until lightly sizzling. Add the sausages and cook for 8 minutes. Add the bacon and cook until crispy. Add the potato bread and cook until it is brown on the outside and soft in the middle. Place tomatoes alongside the bread and cook for several minutes until a little crispy. After 2 to 3 minutes, flip everything over. When everything in done, remove it to a plate and keep it warm while you cook the eggs. Clean the pan and add fresh oil before cooking the eggs. For sunny side up, place a lid on the pan to cook the top to the desired amount of doneness. Place the cooked eggs on the plate with the rest of the meal and enjoy.

Food Trivia

What is *champ*?
A potato mash flavored with shredded scallions which originated in Northern Ireland.

What is a *jacket*?
A potato fried, roasted, baked in the skin, and peeled at the table.

What is *dulse*?
A salty seaweed snack, originally harvested by fishermen to supplement their income when fishing was slack.

What is served at Halloween?
Lough Neagh eel is served fried in chunks with a white onion sauce, It is also smoked and served as a starter.

What is potato bread *farl*?
A dense, earthy flat bread, made with potatoes, flour, and buttermilk, and cooked on a griddle.

What is the history of soda bread *farl*?
It was first baked in nineteenth-century Ireland when local peasants added baking soda to help the dough rise. The result is thick, chunky, soft bread with a fluffy consistency that is best served fried as part of the Ulster Fry or toasted and served with a dollop of butter.

What traditional bread is used to make Paddy's Pizzas?
Soda bread.

What is *wheaten* bread?
A healthy brown bread made with whole-wheat flour, it is delicious toasted with melted cheese or buttered and served with a big bowl of steaming broth.

What is Yellow Man?
A crunchy golden confection often confused with honeycomb and similar in texture, sold at fairs and markets.

What is a vegetable roll?
Thick slices of a fatty meat from the trimmings of brisket and ribs, seasoned with fresh vegetables, usually celery, leek, carrot, and onion.

Customs

Weddings

When the Scots and English arrived and conquered Ireland in the 1600s, there was very little intermarriage between them and the original Irish inhabitants. Today, as many as one-fifth of marriages in Belfast are between a Catholic and a Protestant, though this figure may be exaggerated.

In the past marriage was tied to inheritance. After the potato famine, because farmers felt betrayed by the land, the generations of birthright to family land stopped. Farmers who had small plots wanted to hold on to what they had and were reluctant to subdivide their parcels to hand down to their sons.

Traditionally a father would give his land to one son, not necessarily the oldest. Only the son who received land could take a bride. Often the land was not given until the father reached the age of 70 at which time an old age pension allowed him to bequeath his land. In the meantime the grown children who were not going to inherit land had no place in the home and usually emigrated, many to the US, or looked for work as craftsmen in a neighboring town.

Parents enjoyed a patriarchal status, with the father claiming the best chair near the fire. Historically when parents retired and passed their land to a son, they stopped sleeping in the kitchen and moved to a smaller room in the back of the house where they would display heirlooms and religious pictures that previously were kept in the main hearth area.

Children

Children generally adopt the father's surname. The first name is generally a Christian name, usually the name of a saint.

Traditionally the mother raises younger children. When a boy makes his first communion, generally at age seven, his father rears him alongside his older brothers.

Sprinkling the baby with cake is an Irish tradition. It's popular to use some of the top tier of the family wedding cake to sprinkle over the baby's head at the christening.

Holidays

January 1, New Year's Day
March 17, St. Patrick's Day
Variable date. Good Friday
Variable date. Easter
Variable date. Easter Monday
First Monday in May. May Day
Last Monday in May. Spring Break
July 12. Orangeman's Day
Last Monday in August. Summer Holiday
December 25. Christmas
December 26. Boxer Day
December 31. New Year's Eve

Customs Trivia

Why ring wedding bells?
Superstition says the sound of bells wards off malicious spirits.

What is the modern version of the wedding bell legend?
Brides wear a small bracelet or bell charms.

Why give wedding guests small bells?
To ring to celebrate the newly married couple.

What is the *Claddagh* ring?
A traditional ring widely given by young Irish men to their girlfriends as a gift, and sometimes inherited from a family member.

How is the *Claddagh* ring worn?
Single women traditionally wear the ring on the right hand with the crown in the design facing outward. When in a relationship, the crown is turned inwards, indicating that the lady isn't available.

When is the *Claddagh* ring worn on the left hand?
When the ring is worn on the left hand with the crown pointing outward it means the wearer is engaged. The ring turned inward on that hand means the wearer is married.

Why have a horseshoe at your wedding?
Traditionally brides who carry a horseshoe on their wedding day bring good luck to the occasion and the rest of the marriage.

What do modern brides carry instead of a horseshoe?
Small symbols of the horseshoe, made of silver or porcelain and often tucked away in their flowers.

What was the traditional color of an Irish wedding gown?
Blue, for purity.

What is tying the knot?
This term comes from an old Irish tradition that symbolizes the bond of marriage in the same way as the exchanging of rings. During the ceremony, the couple clasp their hands together and a ribbon, cord, or rope is wound around their joined hands as a symbol of their agreement to spend their lives together.

More Resources

DVDs

Bring Me Back to Old Ireland, DVD, www.Musiccitydirect.com, 2011.
Lakes & Legends of the British Isles: Northern Ireland, DVD, Beckman Studio, 2013.
Music of Northern Ireland, DVD, DPTV Media, 2015.
Wildfowling and Rough Shooting in Ireland, DVD, John Thompson video, 1999.

Books

Cochrane, F. *Northern Ireland: The Reluctant Peace* (Yale University Press, 2013).
DK Publishing. *Back Roads Ireland* (DK Publishing, 2013).

Fletcher, M. *Silver Linings: Travels Around Northern Ireland* (Little, Brown Book Group, 2001).
Mullholland, M. *Northern Ireland: A Very Short Introduction* (Oxford University Press, 2003).
Steves, R. *Rick Steves' Snapshot Northern Ireland* (Avalon Travel Publishing; 2014).

Websites

Arts Council of Northern Ireland: Accessed March 8, 2015, http://www.artscouncil-ni.org/
Northern Ireland Office: Accessed March 8, 2015, https://www.gov.uk/government/organisations/northern-ireland-office
Society of Genealogists of Northern Ireland: Accessed March 8, 2015, http://www.sgni.net/
The Official Visitors Website for Northern Ireland: Accessed March 8, 2015, http://www.discovernorthernireland.com/
Tours of Northern Ireland: Accessed March 8, 2015, http://inroadsireland.com/tours/go-north?gclid=COzx6NvRmMQCFWIV7AodG1YAIQ

Photos

Irish Photos. Accessed March 8, 2015, http://www.freeirishphotos.com/
Northern Ireland: Accessed March 8, 2015, http://www.worldatlas.com/webimage/countrys/europe/ukni.htm
Photos of Northern Ireland: Accessed March 8, 2015, http://www.greatbigcanvas.com/category/scenery-by-region/europe/northern-ireland/?gclid=CKiPuuPTmMQCFRRo7AodszcAtg
Photos of Northern Ireland: Accessed March 8, 2015, http://www.ireland.com/en-us/amazing-places/northern-ireland?gclid=CM2Pp5rTmMQCFSNk7Aod5TAA9g
Pictures of Ireland: Accessed March 8, 2015, http://www.irelandpictures.net/

References

10 Celebrities You Might Not Know Are Irish: Accessed March 7, 2015, http://thefw.com/surprising-irish-celebrities/?trackback=tsmclip

38 Properties in Londonderry: Accessed March 7, 2015, http://www.booking.com/searchresults.en-us.html?aid=318759;label=msn-0zBKDv6hE0YJginwY99Dpw-6302328897;sid=67d1273fe34830b3a4b800c7076086b4;dcid=1;dest_id=-2601896;dest_type=city&;dathm=0

75 Hotels in Belfast: Accessed March 7, 2015, http://www.expedia.com/Hotel-Search#destination=Belfast+%28and+vicinity%29&regionId=6034919&startDate=03%2F08%2F2015&endDate=03%2F11%2F2015&adults=2&selected=1406421

Culture of Northern Ireland: Accessed March 7, 2015, http://www.everyculture.com/No-Sa/Northern-Ireland.html

Facts About Northern Ireland: Accessed March 7, 2015, http://lifestyle.iloveindia.com/lounge/facts-about-northern-ireland-10996.html

Five Old Wedding Traditions You May Not Know About: Accessed March 7, 2015, http://www.irishcentral.com/roots/five-old-irish-wedding-traditions-you-may-not-know-about-photos-221339081-237772511.html

Fun Facts About Ireland: Accessed March 7, 2015, http://www.uniquely-northern-ireland.com/Fun-Facts-About-Ireland.html#sthash.BK0B37OH.dpuf

How to Make the Perfect Ulster Fry: Accessed March 7, 2015, http://www.belfasttelegraph.co.uk/life/recipes/how-to-cook-the-perfect-ulster-fry-29962910.html

Ireland Map Coloring Printout: Accessed March 7, 2015, http://www.enchantedlearning.com/europe/ireland/activity.shtml

Murderpedia: Accessed March 7, 2015, http://www.murderpedia.org/male.B/b/burke-william.htm

Northern Ireland: Accessed March 7, 2015, http://famouswonders.com/europe/northern-ireland/ Accessed March 7, 2015

Northern Ireland Flag Coloring Page: Accessed March 7, 2015, http://www.activityvillage.co.uk/northern-ireland-flag-colouring-page

Pearson Education: Accessed March 7, 2015, http://www.infoplease.com/country/northern-ireland.html?pageno=3

Rootsweb. Ancestry.com: Accessed March 7, 2015, http://rwguide.rootsweb.ancestry.com/irish/famous.html#famous

St. Patrick Centre: Accessed March 7, 2015, http://www.saintpatrickcentre.com/info.php

The Best Bands to Come out of Northern Ireland: Accessed March 7, 2015, http://www.huffingtonpost.co.uk/2013/05/17/top-ten-bands-and-musicians-from-northern-ireland_n_3291118.html

The History of Irish Dance: Accessed March 7, 2015, http://www.irelandseye.com/dance.html

The Official Website of C. S. Lewis: Accessed March 7, 2015, https://www.cslewis.com/us/about-cs-lewis

The Ulster-Scots Society of America: Accessed March 7, 2015, http://www.ulsterscotssociety.com/about_the-roots.html

Traditional Dishes: Accessed March 7, 2015,
   http://www.discovernorthernireland.com/Traditional-Dishes-A1943

Traditional Irish Games for Kids: Accessed March 7, 2015,
   http://www.ehow.com/list_6768361_traditional-irish-games-kids.html

Travel Math United Kingdom: Accessed March 7, 2015,
   http://www.travelmath.com/from/Seattle,+WA/to/Belfast,+United+Kingdom

World Atlas: Accessed March 7, 2015,
   http://www.worldatlas.com/webimage/countrys/europe/northernireland/uknifamous.
   htm

NORWAY

Basics

Geography

Norway is the farthest north of any European country. It is situated in the western part of the Scandinavian Peninsula. It extends about 1,100 miles from the North Sea along the Norwegian Sea to more than 300 miles above the Arctic Circle. Nearly 70 percent of the country is uninhabitable, covered by mountains, glaciers, moors, and rivers. It has an oceanfront of more than 12,000 miles. Galdhø Peak at 8,100 feet is Norway's highest point and the Glomma at 372 miles long is the main river. Norway is slightly larger than New Mexico.

Language

The official languages are Bokmal Norwegian and Nynorsk Norwegian. Minority languages are Sami and Finnish. Sami is an official language in nine municipalities.

History

The history of Norway began with the Norsemen, also known as Vikings, who lived and traveled to the coasts northwest Europe from the eighth to the eleventh centuries. They began as tribes ruled by local chieftains. Olaf II Haraldsson became the first king of Norway in 1015 and began converting the Norwegians to Christianity.

Beginning in 1442, Norway was ruled by Danish kings until 1814 when it was united with Sweden. It remained so until 1905 when the

Norwegian parliament arranged a peaceful separation and invited the Danish King Haakon VII to the Norwegian throne. By treaty with Sweden, all disputes would be settled by arbitration and no fortifications would be erected on the common frontier.

Norway was neutral during World War I. Norway was invaded by the Germans on April 9, 1940, during World War II. King Haakon and his government fled to London and established a government-in-exile. Major Vidkun Quisling, who served as Norway's prime minister during the war, was a Nazi collaborator. Quisling has since become the Norwegian word for traitor. He was executed by the Norwegians on October 24, 1945. The country joined NATO in 1949.

Map and Flag

Norway Coloring Pages: Accessed March 25, 2015,
    http://www.coloring.ws/norway.htm
Norway Flag Printables: Accessed March 25, 2015,
    http://www.activityvillage.co.uk/norway-flag-printables

Travel

Distance

From New York, NY, to Oslo is 3,685 miles. Flight time is 7 hours 52 minutes.

From Chicago, IL, to Oslo is 4,050 miles. Flight time is 8 hours 36 minutes.

From Dallas, TX, to Oslo is 4,850 miles. Flight time is 10 hours 12 minutes.

From Seattle, WA, to Oslo is 4,568 miles. Flight time is 9 hours 38 minutes.

Hotels

Bekkjarvik Gjestgiveri. Located on an island it has hosted guests for more than 300 years. The current owner's son Orjan Johannessen won first place in the 2012 European professional cooking competition and can often be found preparing food for guests.

Canvas Hotel. Located in Telemark, it features a unique hotel experience. Guests stay in one of ten Mongolian-style yurts that have wooden floors, comfortable beds, and outdoor bathtubs to soak in after a day of mountain biking or hiking in the beautiful surrounding countryside.

Hanseatic Hotel. Located in the heart of the UNESCO World Heritage site Bryggen. Small but perfectly formed, this intimate hotel is housed in a wooden building and furnished in sixteenth-century style, giving visitors a feeling for what the town of Bergen was like in its medieval trading days.

Hotel Brosundet. A small boutique hotel with 46 rooms located in Alesund. You can spend the night in the lighthouse overlooking the ocean and have dinner in the hotel's gourmet restaurant featuring freshly caught seafood.

Kviknes Hotel. Located in Balestrand, it been operated by the Kvikne family since 1877. It is built in Swiss chalet style and has a large collection of art and antiques that guests can view.

Landmarks

Geirangerfjord. Located in southwestern Norway, a perfect place to enjoy fishing, kayaking, and hiking along paths by waterfalls. There are lookout points for taking photos of the mountains Dalsnibba and Flydalsjuvet.

Oscarsborg Fortress. Built in 1853 to protect Oslo, it was a site of heavy fighting between Norway and Germany during World War II. It eventually fell to German forces and was used for quartering German soldiers. Tours are available and on special occasions visitors can attend an opera in the courtyard.

Svalbard. A group of islands located between the Arctic Ocean, Barents Sea, Greenland Sea, and the Norwegian Sea, they are the northernmost permanently inhabited spots on the planet. Visitors can see glaciers and mountains, as well as polar bears, caribou, reindeer, polar foxes, whales, seals, and walruses in their natural environment.

Trollstigen Mountain Road. Located in Romsdal in a natural area for hiking, camping, and canoeing along the Istra River. Due to harsh winter weather, the trails usually open in June.

Urnes Stave Church. Located in Ornes, this is one of about 30 surviving stave churches of the 1,300 built in Norway during medieval times. *Stave* refers to a wooden church of post and lintel design. This church was built between the twelfth and thirteenth centuries and is admired for its combination of architecture styles.

Travel Trivia

Where is the deepest lake in Europe?
Hornindalsvatnet, in central Norway, is Europe's deepest lake at 1,686 feet.

Where is Europe's highest waterfall?
Vinnufossen in Norway at 2,822 feet, the sixth tallest in the world.

True or false: Norway has the longest road tunnel in the world.
True. The Lærdal Tunnel is 15.2 miles long.

True or false: Norway has the deepest undersea tunnel in the world.
True. The Eiksund Tunnel is 25,476 feet long and reaches a depth of 942 feet.

True or False: Norway has the longest coastline in Europe.
False: Russia has the longest coastline in Europe. Norway is second.

What kitchen tool was invented in Norway?
The modern cheese slicer was patented in 1925 by Thor Bjørklund.

What spray product was invented in Norway?
The aerosol spray can was invented in 1926 by the chemical engineer Erik Rotheim from Oslo.

Who was Trygve Lie?
The first secretary general of the United Nations. He was from Norway and served from 1946 to 1952.

When did Norway became one of the first countries to establish a Ministry for the Environment?
1972.

What is the official name of Norway?
The Kingdom of Norway.

Why is Norway called the Land of the Midnight Sun?
From late May to late July the sun never completely drops below the horizon in the areas of Norway above the Arctic Circle and other areas have about 20 hours of sunlight a day. This light pattern is the opposite in winter.

What is a troll?
In Norwegian folklore a troll is an ugly, messy, nasty creature that lives in caves or forests and will turn to stone if sunlight hits it.

What is the capitol of Norway?
Oslo.

What office product was invented in Norway?
The paper clip.

True or false: In Norway you must pay an annual fee for owning a television set.
True. The annual fee is about US$300.

True or false: Norwegian newspapers are subsidized by the government.
True.

True or false: Norway's police stations are closed on the weekends.
True.

True or false: Norwegians love to start conversations with strangers.
False: This is considered very rude.

True or false: There is a Doomsday Vault in Norway.
True. The Norwegian Government spent US$7 million on the construction of a doomsday seed vault to preserve plants seeds from around the world.

Who do Norwegians say discovered America?
Viking explorer Leif Erikson in 1003 AD, the first European to set foot on the American continent.

America's Roots

Who was Reidar Fauske Sognnaes?
Born in Bergen, Norway, he became Dean of the Harvard School of Dental Medicine, founding Dean of the UCLA School of Dentistry, and a world-renowned scholar in the field of oral pathology.

Who was Carl Blegen?
An American archaeologist of Norwegian descent famous for his work on the site of Pylos in modern-day Greece and Troy in modern-day Turkey.

Who was Elise M. Boulding?
A Quaker sociologist and author credited as a major contributor to the creation of the academic discipline of Peace and Conflict Studies. She was born in Oslo and came to the US as an infant.

Who was George Bergstrom?
Born in Wisconsin of Norwegian ancestry, he was the architect who designed the Pentagon.

Who was Joachim Goschen Giæver?
A civil engineer who helped with the construction of the framework of the Statue of Liberty. Born in Norway, he came to the US in 1882.

Who is Richard Dean Anderson?
A television and film actor, producer, and composer who is of Norwegian descent.

Who was James Arness?
An actor best known for portraying Marshal Matt Dillon in the television series *Gunsmoke*. His father was of Norwegian ancestry.

Who was James Cagney?
A stage and film actor born in New York of Norwegian descent.

Who was Bob Fosse?
An actor, dancer, musical theater choreographer, director, screenwriter, film editor, and film director who was born in Illinois of Norwegian descent.

Who is Linda Evans?
An actress known for her roles in *The Big Valley* and *Dynasty*. She was born in Connecticut and her paternal great-grandmother was born in Hedmark, Norway.

Who was Reuben Trane?
The founder of the heating and air-conditioning company Trane. He was born in Wisconsin of Norwegian descent.

Who was Conrad Hilton?
The founder of the Hilton Hotels chain. Born in New Mexico, he was of Norwegian descent.

Who was Jafet Lindeberg?
A gold prospector and co-founder of the city of Nome, Alaska. He was born in Troms County, Norway, and came to the US in 1897.

Who was Charles M. Schulz?
A cartoonist and creator of the comic strip *Peanuts*. Of Norwegian descent, he was born in Minneapolis, MN.

Who was Sally Ride?
An astronaut and the first American woman to go to space. She was born in California and was of Norwegian descent.

Sports and Games

Sports

The most popular sport in Norway is football, which Americans call soccer. However, what is unique is the country's financial support of public involvement in sports. Sporting organizations for adults and children receive 90 to 95 percent of their funding from the government. With an emphasis on sports for all, sporting programs are equally funded for men and women.

Over 40 percent of adults take part in physical sporting activities. There are sporting organizations for children in every city and the emphasis for youth under age 10 is on participation and mental health rather than winning.

Norway is the birthplace of skiing and has 18,600 miles of marked ski trails. Winter weather allows for perfect skiing conditions from December to April and sometimes even through May in the higher elevations.

Norway is best known for its cross-country skiing. There are many resorts and schools where the emphasis is on skiing for pleasure.

Other sports include boxing, wrestling, speed-skating, curling, cycling, dancing, sledge-dog racing, handball, karate, orienteering, canoeing, rowing, sailing, shooting, weight-lifting, and swimming.

Sports Trivia

Who were Birkebeinars?
In 1296 members of this rebellious political faction saved the Norwegian prince Haakon Haakonsen by carrying the baby 55 miles. The route they took became a cross-country ski track where 6000 people race every year.

Who was Sondre Norheim?
He designed the Telemark ski and combined ordinary skiing with jumping and slalom.

When did the first skis arrive in America?
The first modern Norwegian skis were brought to the US in 1825.

True or false: Norway is the only country that has never lost a soccer game to Brazil.
True.

True or false: The word ski comes from Norway.
True. It comes from the Old Norse word *skíð* which means stick of wood or ski.

True or false: Norway holds the most Olympic medals in winter sports.
True, 303 medals as of 2012.

When was the rat-trap ski binding invented?
In 1927 by the Norwegian Bror With.

Who is Audun Endestad?
A Norwegian cross-country skier, author, and field guide.

Who was Alf Engen?
A skier and skiing school owner/teacher who set several ski jumping world records in the 1930s.

Who was Sonja Henie?
A Norwegian figure skater, actress, and film star.

Game

Gurka is a popular Norwegian card game.
Number of players. Five
Materials. A table and a deck of 52 cards with the jokers removed.
To play. For the first hand, five cards are dealt to each player. Subsequently the number of cards dealt is equal to the value of the card held by the loser of the previous hand, with a maximum deal of seven cards each.

In the first round the dealer plays first. In subsequent rounds the person who played the lowest card in the previous round deals the next hand. If two or more persons played the lowest card, the first to do so deals the next hand. The dealer may discard some cards, keeping at least two, and draw replacements. If the dealer does this, each of the other players has the option to exchange the same number of cards as the dealer or play with their original hand.

Winner. The player who first reaches a total card value of 21. The value of kings, queens, jacks, and aces is 11 each.

CHFI benefits. Cognitive, language, speech, hand and eye coordination, math, and physical skills of voluntary body movement, muscle force, and mobility of joints.

Music and Dance

Music

Norway has a long unbroken folk music tradition passed from generation to generation. Norwegian folk music, both vocal and instrumental, is usually performed by soloists.

Instrumental music is most commonly played on the fiddle, especially the Hardanger fiddle which is considered the national instrument of Norway. The Hardanger fiddle is a violin with four or five sympathetic strings which is beautifully decorated and is constructed somewhat differently from an ordinary violin.

In addition to the musical traditions of Southern and Middle-Norway, the North also holds treasures in the form of Sami folk music which includes a powerful chanting vocal style called *joik*.

The Sami are an indigenous people of Northern Europe across four countries: Norway, Sweden, Russia, and Finland. The Sami population is estimated at 75,000.

Joik themes range from the life of the singer to tales of animals, people, places, feelings, and hopes. A traditional *joik* is often about people smirking, admiring, pitying, proposing marriage, and seducing. Thus a *joik* is a way for a singer to process and release emotions.

Traditional musical instruments include the *bukkehorn* which is a goat horn, the *harpeleik* which is a chorded zither, the *langeleik* which is a box dulcimer, the *lur* which is trumpet-like, the *seljefløyte* which is a willow flute, the *tungehorn* and *melhus* which are clarinet-like, and the *munnharpe* which is a jaw harp.

Music Videos

Norwegian Folk Music: Accessed March 25, 2015,
    https://www.youtube.com/watch?v=zJsvzFX8MJ0
Norwegian Folk Song: Accessed March 25, 2015.
    https://www.youtube.com/watch?v=mB71Sqh9iB8
Norway Folk Dance Music: Accessed March 25, 2015,
    https://www.youtube.com/watch?v=-98vYMKahTc

Dance

The history of dance in Norway began with song dances that told the tales of heroes. In the eighteenth century the increasing popularity of musical instruments began the decline of song dance as did the influences of European dances such as the polka and waltz. The accordion, flute, and zither ingrained themselves into the culture along with the movements meant to accompany them.

In the 1880s musician Hulda Garborg discovered that earlier folk songs were meant to be dances. She made up steps to go with the songs. In 1902 she compared her dances to those of the Faroe Islands where song dances were still performed. Garborg put the two styles together and began teaching the dance throughout the country.

Folk dances in Norway are regionally influenced. Every section has a signature dance and its own costume called *bunad*. Each village might have its own version of the dance to any given song. Formerly only locals knew their own dances but thanks to the oral and written record of the dances, now most village dances are known across the country.

All of these traditions are nurtured by two annual national competitions which celebrate this cultural heritage, the National Folk Dance Music Festival and the National Contest for Traditional Music. The Norwegian Traditional Music and Dance Association, founded in 1987, advances the cause of folk dance and music, ensuring that the old traditions will continue into the future intact and enjoyed.

Dance Videos

Norwegian Folk Dancing: Accessed March 25, 2015,
    https://www.youtube.com/watch?v=BihYMeir2YM
Norwegian National Day: Accessed March 25, 2015,
    https://www.youtube.com/watch?v=Hs8n-280tzg
Traditional Norwegian Dance: Accessed March 25, 2015,
    https://www.youtube.com/watch?v=9BXbL0m6iq8

Music and Dance Trivia

Name some popular Norwegian singers.
Adjagas, Majorstuen, Annbjørg Lien, Mari Boine, and Unni Løvlid.

True or false: *The Three Billy Goats Gruff* is a Norwegian fairy tale.
True. The author is unknown.

Name classical composers from Norway.
Georg von Bertouch, Johan Daniel Berlin, Edvard Grieg, and Johan Henrik Berlin.

Who was Ole Bull?
A fiddler who was the first Norwegian musician known outside the country.

When was the Bergen Philharmonic Orchestra founded?
1765.

When was Norway's most popular orchestra founded?
The Oslo Philharmonic Orchestra was founded in 1919.

How old is choir singing in Norway?
It dates back to the twelfth century.

What is Norway's most popular country-style band?
Hellbellies.

What is *dansbandsmusik*?
Dance music played by classical, electric, bass, and steel guitars, drum, saxophone, accordion, and keyboard.

What is *Insomnia*?
A festival of innovative electronic music held annually in Tromso.

Food

Brunost, a brown cheese sliced thin and eaten on bread is a staple in the Norwegian diet. A typical breakfast consists of coffee, bread, flatbread, or crisp bread, pickled or smoked fish, cold meats, boiled eggs, and milk products such as cheese, butter, yogurt, and various types of sour milk. Breakfast is often more substantial than lunch.

The noon meal or *lunsj* is usually an open-faced sandwich of bread, cheese, or cold meat, perhaps accompanied by a piece of fruit and coffee. The late meal of the day can be fish and meat, including pork, beef, lamb, chicken, and whale, and boiled potatoes, usually served with gravy or melted butter. Root vegetables such as carrots often supplement potatoes. Beer or wine is occasionally consumed in the evening.

The Norwegians are not immune to fast food. Pizza and hamburgers are popular occasional meals and often are served at restaurants. Cafés and cafeterias serve open-faced sandwiches of cold meats, smoked fish, or cheese as well as simple but substantial meals of meat or fish and boiled potatoes.

Chinese, Indian, and other ethnic restaurants can be found as Norwegian cuisine has become more diversified and international. Although the consumption of fats and fish has gone down in the last 20 years, the consumption of meat has never been higher.

Recipe

Fyrstekake. This classic dessert is also known as Royal Cake or Prince's Cake but is closer to an American pie. Serves 8-12.

Ingredients.

For the crust:

2¼ cups flour

¾ cup powdered sugar

14 tablespoons cold unsalted butter cut into 3/4-inch cubes

1 egg.

For the filling:

1¾ cups slivered almonds

1 cup sugar

1 tablespoon butter

1 egg yolk

1 whole egg

1/4 cup whipping cream.

For the topping:

1 egg yolk mixed with 1 tablespoon water

Preparation. To make the crust, pulse flour, powdered sugar, and butter in a food processor until crumbly. Add the egg and form into dough. Turn the dough out onto a piece of plastic wrap, cover it well, and refrigerate for at least two hours.

Grease an 8" or 9" tart pan with a removable base. Roll out the dough on a lightly floured surface to about ⅛" thick. Place in the tart pan and work it evenly into the crease and up the sides. Put the pan and the remaining dough in the refrigerator for 30 minutes while you prepare the filling. Preheat the oven to 335 degrees F.

In the food processor chop the almonds until fine, then add the sugar and pulse until combined. Melt the butter and stir it into the almond and sugar mixture along with the egg yolk, egg, and whipping cream. Process to blend and then pour the filling into the prepared crust.

Roll out the remaining dough on a lightly floured surface. Cut the dough into thin strips and arrange them in a lattice or crisscross pattern on top of the filling.

Mix the remaining egg yolk with a tablespoon of water and brush this over the top of the cake. Bake for approximately 40 minutes until golden.

Food Trivia

How is the brown cheese *brunost* made?
The water left over from the regular goat cheese making process is evaporated.

What do Norwegians take every day for health?
A spoonful of cod liver oil.

What food do most Norwegians eat daily?
Kaviar, a form of mashed cod.

True or false: Norwegian food stores are closed on Sunday.
True. Only kiosks and gas stations may sell food on a Sunday.

Where can you buy wine and liquor?
Only in a *Vinmonopol* store. Drunk drivers are jailed for 30 days, lose their license, and pay a fine of 10 percent of their annual income.

True or false: Many Norwegians buy their food in Sweden.
True. Prices are a lot lower in Sweden.

What frozen food do Norwegians love?
Frozen pizza.

What seafood dish is considered a delicacy?
Lutefisk, although not everyone agrees.

True or False: The government subsidizes Norwegian farmers.
True.

True or false: The Norwegian government controls farm production.
True. The production of milk and meat is regulated.

Customs

Weddings

The majority of weddings in Norway are much smaller in size than most American weddings. The bride and groom invite those family and friends that are closest to them and children are generally not invited.

A traditional Norwegian wedding procession begins with fiddle players leading the way followed by the bride and the groom. Next in order came the parents of the couple, bridesmaids, ring bearer, flower girls, with guests coming last. In some areas of the country, the groom and other male guests ride in front of the women. The bride would always have the best horse, usually light-colored.

Some wedding parties arrived at the church or ceremony location by foot, carriage, or boat. What mattered most was the correct line-up of the procession.

Only one attendant stood on each side of the bride and groom during the ceremony, along with the flower girl and ring bearer.

After the ceremony, a dinner of several courses is held, lasting several hours and including songs and toasts to the bride and groom. The toastmaster introduces each person who wants to speak and keeps the order of the toasts: father of the bride, the groom, the bride, maid of honor, best man, groom's father, bride's mother, groom's mother, grandparents/godparents, friends, and finally the *Thank You for the Meal* speech.

At the end of the meal, the wedding cake is cut and guests can also help themselves to a variety of cakes, coffee, and an after-dinner drink. The bride and groom can ask friends and family to supply extra cakes for the cake table. Some favorites are almond cake, cheesecake, and chocolate cake.

The bride and groom have the first dance. After a period of dancing, guests will be served *nattmat*, night food — sausages, soup with bread, or sandwiches.

Children

Infants sleep in their own cribs and often in prams outdoors as the Norwegians believe fresh air is good for the baby's health. Modern mothers believe in breastfeeding on demand and carry infants close to their chests in slings. Norwegians also believe that playing outdoors is good for children.

Daycare is provided beginning at age one year, however many parents wait until the child is an older toddler.

Confirmation in the church is an important rite of passage and social event. The ceremony is followed by a party to which neighbors and relatives are invited and where young girls are given a *bunad*, a traditional folk costume.

Holidays

January 1. New Year's Day
Variable date. Maundy Thursday
Variable date. Good Friday
Variable date. Easter
Variable date. Easter Monday
May 1. Labor Day
Variable date. Ascension Day
Variable date. Whit Sunday
Variable date. Whit Monday
May 17. Constitution Day
December 25. Christmas Day
December 26. Boxing Day
December 31. New Year's Eve

Customs Trivia

What is a traditional gift for the newly married couple?
A gift to use in their new home.

What do guests do before leaving the wedding?
Stand and shake hands with the groom.

What do Norwegians do when entering the home of the newly married couple?
Remove their shoes. This is frequently done when visiting anyone to avoid getting winter slush on the hosts' floors.

Where are children not accepted?
At evening social gatherings.

Why should a pregnant woman avoid looking at rabbits?
Superstition says the unborn child would develop a cleft lip.

Why do you never set sail among seals?
Nordic legends says to do so will bring your death.

What happens if you place your bag on the floor?
You will be poor.

Why shouldn't a girl sit at the corner of the table?
Sitting there will keep you from marrying for seven years.

What happens if a boy sits at the corner of a table?
He will find a wife.

What happens if a man wipes his hands on the apron of an unmarried woman?
He will fall in love with her, but if he wipes his hands on his wife's apron he can expect bad luck and quarrels.

More Resources

DVDs

7 Days Norway, DVD. Travel Video Store, 2007.
Nature Wonders Lofoten Norway, DVD. Amazon Instant Video, 2007.
Norway From the Land of Vikings, DVD. Travel Video Store, 2010.
Passport to Adventure Enchanting, Natural Norway, DVD. Travel Video Store, 2009.
Richard Bangs' Adventures with Purpose: Norway, DVD. Blue Ray, 2009.

Books

DK Publishing. *DK Eyewitness Travel Guide: Norway* (DK Publishing, 2014).
Ham, A. *Lonely Planet Norway* (Lonely Planet, 2011).

Lee, P. *The Rough Guide to Norway* (Rough Guide, 2012).
Rutledge, L. and Rutledge, P. *Experience Norway* (CreateSpace Independent Publishing Platform, 2015).
Steves, R. *Rick Steves' Snapshot Norway* (Avalon Travel Publishing, 2012).

Websites

Embassy of the United States Oslo Norway: Accessed March 25, 2015, http://norway.usembassy.gov/
Flag of Norway: Accessed March 25, 2015, http://www.norden.org/en/fakta-om-norden-1/the-nordic-flags/norways-flag
Government.no: Accessed March 25, 2015, https://www.regjeringen.no/en/id4/
Norway Powered by Nature: Accessed March 25, 2015, http://www.visitnorway.com/us/
Norway The Official Website in the US: Accessed March 25, 2015, http://www.norway.org/

Photos

A Bird's Eye View of Fjord, Norway: Accessed March 25, 2015, http://onebigphoto.com/most-beautiful-landscape-photos-of-norway/
Most Beautiful Landscape Photos of Norway: Accessed March 25, 2015, http://onebigphoto.com/most-beautiful-landscape-photos-of-norway/
Norway In 50 Stunning Photos: Accessed March 25, 2015, http://www.pxleyes.com/blog/2012/07/norway-photography/
Norway photos: Accessed March 25, 2015, http://travel.nationalgeographic.com/travel/countries/norway-photos/
Photos of Norway: Accessed March 25, 2015, http://www.studentsoftheworld.info/infopays/photos/pic.php?CP=N
OR

References

Countries and Their Culture. Norway: Accessed March 25, 2015, http://www.everyculture.com/No-Sa/Norway.html

Famous Landmarks in Norway: Accessed March 25, 2015,
    http://traveltips.usatoday.com/names-famous-landmarks-norway-57732.html
Folk World Scene from Inside: Accessed March 25, 2015,
    http://folkworld.de/9/e/sami.html
Funny Facts about Norway: Accessed March 25, 2015,
    http://funnynorwayfacts.blogspot.com
Hotels in Fjord, Norway: Accessed March 21, 2015,
    http://www.dehistoriske.com/romantic-holiday/hotel-brosundet/
Fyrstekake, an All-Time Favorite Norwegian Dessert: Accessed March 25, 2015,
    http://www.outside-oslo.com/2013/08/05/fyrstekake-an-all-time-favorite-norwegian-
    dessert/
Gurka: Accessed March 25, 2015, http://www.pagat.com/last/cucumber.html#agurk
Interesting Facts about Norway: Accessed March 25, 2015,
    http://www.eupedia.com/norway/trivia.shtml
Norway: Accessed March 21, 2015,
    http://www.infoplease.com/country/norway.html?pageno=2
Norway Facts for Kids: Accessed March 25, 2015,
    http://www.sciencekids.co.nz/sciencefacts/countries/norway.html
Norway Powered by Nature: Accessed March 21, 2015
    http://www.visitnorway.com/us/media--press/ideas-and-features/truly-unique-
    places-to-stay/
Norwegian Americans: Accessed March 25, 2015,
    http://www.ask.com/wiki/List_of_Norwegian_Americans?o=2800&qsrc=999&ad=d
    oubleDown&an=apn&ap=ask.com
Norwegian Wedding Customs: Accessed March 25, 2015,
    https://www.ingebretsens.com/culture/weddings/norw-wed-tradition
Skiing in Norway: Accessed March 25, 2015,
    http://www.frommers.com/destinations/norway/254439#sthash.GS4lmfOX.dpbs
Sports in Norway: Accessed March 25, 2015,
    http://www.reisenett.no/norway/facts/nature_outdoors/sports.html
Superstitions: Accessed March 25, 2015,
    http://www.philbrodieband.com/jokes_superstitions.htm
Ten Best Place to Visit in Norway: Accessed March 25, 2015,
    http://www.touropia.com/best-places-to-visit-in-norway/
The History of Norwegian Folk Dance: Accessed March 25, 2015,
    http://www.ehow.com/about_6469471_history-norwegian-folk-dance.html
This is Music from Norway: Accessed March 25, 2015,
    http://www.musicfromnorway.com/default.aspx?norwegian=album&music=-104
Travelmath Norway: Accessed March 21, 2015,
    http://www.travelmath.com/from/Oslo,+Norway/to/Chicago,+IL

SCOTLAND

Basics

Geography

Scotland is located north of England on an island bounded by the North Sea on the east and the Atlantic Ocean on the west. It is divided into two regions, the Highlands and the Lowlands, The Highlands in the northwest half of the country are mountainous with many steep peeks and deep valleys, The Lowlands are rolling hills and farmland. It has over 790 islands, of which 130 are inhabited. Scotland is known for over 600 square miles of *lochs* which are fresh water lakes.

Language

The official language is English. However, 1,000 years ago the majority of the population spoke Scottish Gaelic. Today about 1.4 percent of the population speak Scottish Gaelic. There is a movement to re-introduce the language, which is taught in some preschools and kindergartens. Scots, which is now considered a dialect of English, was the official language beginning around 1300 and lasting until 1707 when English was made the official language by law.

History

The earliest recorded history of Scotland dates to the arrival of the Romans in 1 AD, resulting in fierce fighting between native inhabitants and the Romans. By 3 AD the Romans had left the country.

In 5 AD northwest Scotland, what is today Northern Ireland, was invaded by the Gaels who established the Kingdom of Dalriada. At the same time the Angles conquered and organized the Anglo-Saxon kingdom of Bernicia in the south.

Both kingdoms fell at the end of the eighth century when Scotland was invaded by the Vikings. Warriors united in the ninth century to form the Kingdom of Scotland.

Fighting for power with invaders from Norway and England continued through the thirteenth century until Scottish landowner Sir William Wallace led a defeat of the English army at the Battle of Stirling Bridge in 1297. In 1305 Wallace was captured in Robroyston, near Glasgow, and handed over to King Edward I of England who had him hanged, drawn, and quartered for high treason. In 1314 Robert the Bruce inflicted a significant defeat on the English at the Battle of Bannockburn.

The Battle of Flodden Field between the Scots led by King James IV and English forces began on the afternoon of September 9, 1513, and by nightfall the Scottish forces had suffered a decisive defeat as well as the loss of their King.

Mary, Queen of Scots, spent only a few years on the Scottish throne before being forced to abdicate to her son James VI. Queen Mary escaped to England to seek help from her cousin Queen Elizabeth I but would never see Scotland again. She was held prisoner in a succession of English castles for over 18 years before being beheaded for her part in a plot to take the English throne.

In 1603, after the death of Elizabeth I of England, James VI of Scotland succeeded to the English throne as James I of England. In 1707 the Acts of Union formally united Scotland with England and Wales as Great Britain.

Map and Flag

Create a map: Accessed March 11, 2015, http://www.coloring-
    pictures.net/drawings/Scotland/Map-of-Scotland.php
Create the flag: Accessed March 11, 2015,
    http://www.coloring.ws/scotland.htm

Travel

Distance

Distance from New York, NY, to Edinburgh is 3,267 miles. Flight time is 7 hours 2 minutes.

Distance from Chicago, IL, to Edinburgh is 3,713 miles. Flight time is 7 hours 56 minutes.

Distance from Dallas, TX, to Edinburgh is 4,517 miles. Flight time is 9 hours 32 minutes.

Distance from Seattle, WA, to Edinburgh is 4,481 miles. Flight time is 9 hours 28 minutes.

Hotels

Ackergill Tower. Located in Wick in a historic building, it offers aroma therapy services to guests. There are a restaurant and a garden on the property.

Glencoe House. Located in Glencoe, Ballachulish, surrounded by mountains, and within nine miles of Glen Coe Visitor Centre, The Ice Factor, and Atlas Brewery. Guests are offered free made-to-order daily breakfasts.

Grand Central Hotel. Located at 99 Gordon Street, Glasgow, in an iconic building where guests can enjoy afternoon tea under the domed ceiling and chandelier at Champagne Central and try Scottish dishes in the Tempus Restaurant. Previous guests at the hotel included John Fitzgerald Kennedy.

Inverlochy Castle. Located at Torlundy Fort William in the historical district 1.2 miles from the Ben Nevis Distillery and within 3 miles of Neptune's Staircase and Leanachan Forest. It provides guests with free rides to the local train station.

The George Hotel. Located at 19-20 George Street in Edinburgh, a block from Princes Street and a quarter mile from the National Gallery. It features an oyster bar.

Landmarks

Cairngorms National Park. Here you can explore vast forests filled with wildlife, enjoy some of the best hillwalking in the country, and ski down snow-covered mountains. It is home to 55 mountain summits and five of the UK's six highest mountains.

Edinburgh. The capitol of Scotland, built on seven hills as is the city of Rome, Italy.

Forth Bridge. This cantilever bridge, which is 120 years old, is considered a marvel of engineering, the first bridge in the United Kingdom to be made of steel. In 1964 it was the fourth largest bridge in the world.

Hadrian's Wall. A stone wall built about 2000 years ago by the Romans to keep out the Picts.

Loch Lomond. The largest lake in Scotland, at 24 square miles.

Loch Ness. A large lake that said to be the home of the Loch Ness Monster, a mysterious water creature with a large head and serpent body reportedly seen by several witnesses over the centuries but never scientifically proven to exist.

Travel Trivia

Who was Sir Robert Watson-Watt?
Considered by many to be the inventor of radar, in 1936 he became superintendent of a new establishment under the British Air Ministry where his work resulted in the design and installation of aircraft detection and tracking stations.

Who was Adam Smith?
Regarded as the father of modern economics, in 1776 he wrote *An Inquiry into the Nature and Causes of the Wealth of Nations* which states the doctrine that labor is the true source of a nation's wealth. He championed individual enterprise and argued for free trade.

Who was Alexander Fleming?
A Scottish bacteriologist whose discovery of penicillin in 1928 started the antibiotic revolution and won him the Nobel Prize.

Who was Kirkpatrick MacMillan?
A blacksmith at Courthill Smithy in Keir Mill, Dumfriesshire, he invented the wheel-propelled bicycle in 1839.

Who was Scott James Chalmers?
The inventor of adhesive postage stamps in 1837 which made mail service more efficient. He made one-penny and two-penny versions.

What is Skara Brae?
Located on the island of Orkney, it is the most complete Neolithic village in Europe and has the oldest building in Britain, dating about 3100 BC.

What is Aberdeen Harbour Board?
Great Britain's oldest recorded business, founded in 1136.

What is The University of St. Andrews?
Founded in 1413, it is the third oldest university in the UK after Oxford and Cambridge. It welcomed Britain's first female student in 1862. The world's first students' union came into existence at St. Andrews in 1882, while the world's oldest students' union building is purpose-built Teviot Row at Edinburgh University, built in 1889.

What is Shores Porters Society in Aberdeen?
Founded in 1498, it is the world's oldest transport company.

When was the Bank of Scotland founded?
In 1695, making it the oldest surviving bank in the UK. It was also the first bank in Europe to print its own banknotes.

Who was William Paterson?
The instigator and a co-founder of the Bank of England.

What is famous about the town of Sanqhar?
The post office at Sanquhar, established in 1712, is the oldest working post office in the world. The town also has the world's oldest curling society, formed in 1774 with 60 members.

What is the Encyclopædia Britannica?
The world's oldest surviving encyclopedia, first published between 1768 and 1771 in Edinburgh.

Who was William Murdoch?
A Scottish engineer who in 1794 built the first house to be lit by gas.

Who was Henry Duncan?
Founder of the world's first commercial savings bank at Ruthwell, near Dumfries, in 1810.

True or false: Edinburgh was the first city in the world with its own fire brigade, in 1824.
True.

What is the Open Championship?
The oldest of the four major golf championships, it was first played in 1860 at Prestwick Golf Club in Ayrshire.

What periodical was founded in 1917 in New York by Scottish-born journalist Bertie Charles Forbes?
Forbes Magazine.

Where is the oldest military air base in the world?
The RAF Leuchars in Fife was established in 1908 and is the oldest continuously operating military air base in the world.

True or false: A Scottish criminal trial may end with a verdict of guilty, not guilty, or not proven.
True.

America's Roots

Who was James Stewart?
An actor and the first movie star to enter the armed service in World War II, he became a Brigadier General in the US Air Force Reserve and earned a Distinguished Flying Cross. He received a Kennedy Center Honor in 1983. He was born in Pennsylvania and his father was of Scottish ancestry.

Who was Sam Houston?
He was elected to Congress in 1823 and was commander in chief of the Texas armies in 1833. In 1836 he defeated Mexico and won independence for Texas. He returned to Congress in 1845 as a Texas senator and served as governor of Texas in 1859. Born in Virginia, he was of Scottish descent.

Who was Johnny Cash?
A singer, songwriter and actor who was inducted into the Country Hall of Fame, Rock and Roll Hall of Fame, and Gospel Music Hall of Fame. *The Johnny Cash Show* aired on television from 1969 to 1971. He served as a staff sergeant in the US Air Force. As a Biblical scholar, he wrote the book *Man in White*. He was born in Arkansas and was of Scottish descent.

Who was Washington Irving?
The author of *Rip Van Winkle* and *The Legend of Sleepy Hollow*, he was also a lawyer and US ambassador to Spain from 1842 to 1846. His parents were Scottish immigrants.

Who was James Monroe?
The fifth president of the United States, he served two terms, wrote the Monroe Doctrine proclaiming independence from European interference in American policy, and purchased Florida from Spain in 1819. He had Scottish ancestors.

Who is Donald Trump?
The billionaire real estate developer whose mother Mary Anne MacLeod hails from Stornoway where she was born in 1912 to fisherman and crofter William MacLeod and his wife Catherine.

Who is Laura-Jean Reese Witherspoon?
An actress and a descendant of Scottish-born John Witherspoon, a signer of the US Declaration of Independence who was born in Gifford, Yester, East Lothian, in 1723 and emigrated to the United States in 1768. He was the only clergyman and college principal to sign the declaration.

Who is Jennifer Aniston?
An actress whose mother Nancy Dow is of Scottish descent.

Who was Elvis Presley?
A singer and actor whose family tree goes back to the Aberdeenshire village of Lonmay, near Fraserburgh. Andrew Presley, whose parents married in Lonmay in 1713, emigrated to the United States of America in 1745 with eventual roots linking him to Elvis' parents who married in 1933 and later gave birth to the world's arguably most famous musician.

Who is Joni Mitchell?

A singer and songwriter who is of Scottish and Irish heritage. Her work is highly respected both by critics and fellow musicians. *Rolling Stone* magazine called her "one of the greatest songwriters ever." She is most famous for her 1970s hit *Big Yellow Taxi*.

Who was Patrick Henry?

A governor of Virginia and a freedom fighter during the American Revolutionary war. He was born in Virginia to parents of Scottish descent.

Who was General Hugh Mercer?

A member of the American Colonial Army during the Seven Years War and a general during American Revolutionary War. He had earlier been in the Battle of Culloden during the Jacobite Rebellion in Scotland. He was born in Scotland and became a close friend of General George Washington.

Who was John Paul Jones?

When John Paul Jones, a Scot, raised the US Stars and Stripes flag on his ship the USS Ranger, the flag was recognized by a foreign power, France, for the first time. Jones is also known as the father of the US Navy.

Who was General Douglas McArthur?

Commander of the US forces in the Pacific theater of operations during World War II. He was born in Arkansas and was of Scottish descent.

Who was General George S. Patton?

The four-star US Army General known as "Blood and Guts," he was a descendant of American Revolutionary War patriot General Hugh Mercer on his mother's side. He had Scottish ancestors.

Sports and Games

Sports

A number of internationally popular sports were invented in Scotland, including golf, rugby, and tennis. Other sports are also rooted in Scotland's history, such as hockey which originated from *shinty*, curling, and, of course, the Scottish Highland Games.

Football is one of the nation's most popular spectator sports. The Scotsman William McGregor established the first English football league and it was in Scotland in 1872 that the first international match was played, in Partick, Glasgow, where England and Scotland drew 0-0.

Traditional Scottish sports, such as tossing the caber, hammer throwing, tug o' war, and cross-country running, are celebrated at more than 60 Scottish Highland Games events across the country every year. Providing a host of fun for spectators and participants alike, the Highland Games are a major part of Scotland's summer sporting agenda.

Sports Trivia

Who banned golf?
The first written reference to golf was in 1457 by King James II of Scotland who banned golf and football in an Act of Parliament on the grounds that they interfered with his subjects' archery practice. Historians believe the game was played much earlier.

How was the original game of golf played?
Called *gowf* in 1457, golf was originally played on a course of 22 holes and was first reduced to 18 holes at the Royal and Ancient Golf Club of St. Andrews in 1764.

What is the oldest Royal golf club in Scotland?
The Royal Perth Golfing Society. Royal Perth was granted its Royal title in 1833. The Royal and Ancient Golf Club received its title in 1834 and Royal Musselburgh followed in 1876.

When were the rules of golf first written down?
The first 13 Rules of Golf were written in 1744 for the Annual Challenge for the Silver Club played for by the Honourable Company of Edinburgh Golfers.

What are golf links?
A stretch of land near the coast characterized by undulating terrain, often associated with dunes and infertile sandy soil.

What is the Highland Football League?
Based primarily in the north of Scotland but also incorporating teams from the northeast lowlands, it is regarded as one of the best associations in Scotland.

Who did Scotland play in the first international rugby match?
The world's first international rugby match was played at Raeburn Place, Edinburgh, on March 27, 1871, against England.

When was the world's first international football competition?
The world's first international football match, Scotland versus England, was held at Hamilton Crescent in Glasgow on November 30, 1872.

True or false: Scotland once had the world's largest sports stadium.
True. From the time of its completion in 1903 until 1950, Hampden Park in Glasgow was the biggest stadium in the world with a capacity in excess of 100,000.

When did the Glasgow Celtic become the first British football club to win the European Cup?
In 1967 when they beat Inter Milan.

Game

Lawn Bowling. Usually played outdoors but adaptable for use indoors, this is a skill game that involves rolling 5" balls called *bowls*. The goal is to roll a *bowl* closest to the target ball, a small white ball called a *jack*. The *bowl* is slightly flattened on one side, causing it to travel a curved path that creates the challenge of the game.

Number of players. Two teams of one to four players each.

Materials. Six 6" diameter soft balls of varied colors, a white aisle cloth or white paper 10' by 3' in size, two kitchen floor mats or similar mats to be placed at both ends of the cloth/paper to secure the ends.

To play. Each team has one bowl. The playing area, called a rink, measures 120 square feet. A rubber mat is placed at the starting end of the rink and the jack is placed in the center. Players take turns rolling their ball toward the jack. The player must keep one foot on the mat when releasing the ball.

Modified for residents who can stand and roll the ball: Use a runner or white drawing paper as the court with kitchen floor mats to secure either end of the court. Small toss balls serve as the bowls and a black ball as the jack.

Winner. The person whose ball comes closest to the jack.

ICHI benefits. Voluntary control of movement, mobility of joints, muscle tone, and mental functions of language.

Music and Dance

Music

Scotland's musical traditions began with the bagpipe, Scotland's national instrument, which seems to have always been part of the culture. The bagpipe is used in pipe bands, traditional folk and ceilidh bands, solo performances, by buskers, and as an accompaniment to Highland dancing. The distinctive sound is synonymous with Scotland as are the myths of its history.

One myth is that the bagpipe was banned by a 1746 proscription act in which the instrument was never actually mentioned.

Legend has it that James Reid, who was hung after the 1745 rebellion, was judged guilty of inciting riot or mutiny by playing his bagpipes. This myth led the way for Scottish romanticists to claim that he was hung because he was a piper and that his pipe became a "war pipe" or "an instrument of war." However, the truth is that players of fifes, horns, and drums were hung during the reign of Henry VI who punished by death anyone who incited a riot or started a mutiny with a musical instrument.

Some believe that before 1700, a clan piper was one of the most important people in clan society, second only to the chief. The reality is he was usually an illiterate domestic servant.

Scotland is the birthplace of the New Year's Eve standard *Auld Lang Syne*. The lyrics were written by Robert Burns in 1788. The phrase "Auld Lang Syne" means "good old days" and is meant to celebrate the kindness and fellowship of family and friends in days gone by:

Should auld acquaintance be forgot
And never brought to mind?
Should auld acquaintance be forgot,

And days o' auld lang syne!

For auld lang syne, my dear
For auld lange syne,
We'll tak a cup o' kindness yet
For auld lang syne!

Music Videos

Auld Lang Syne: Accessed February 2013,
    http://www.youtube.com/watch?v=AItlCyEX9nc&feature=related
National Anthem of Scotland Flower of Scotland Bagpipe: Accessed
    March 8, 2015, https://www.youtube.com/watch?v=aLrzQu7FsEo
Scotland The Brave 51st Highland Division: Accessed March 8, 2015,
    https://www.youtube.com/watch?v=umzRoqtWvrA

Dance

Legend says that Highland dances began because kings and clan chiefs used the Highland Games as a means to select their best men at arms. The discipline required to perform the Highland dances allowed men to demonstrate their strength, stamina, and agility.

The first documented evidence of intricate war-dances being performed to "the wailing music of bagpipes" was in 1285. Historians also believe that Scottish mercenaries performed a sword dance before the Swedish King John III at a banquet held at Stockholm Castle in 1573. The dance was part of a plot to assassinate the king and the weapons necessary to complete the dastardly deed just happened to be a natural prop for the festivities. Fortunately for the king, the signal was never given to implement the plan.

In 1746 a law was passed and enforced in the City of London which made the carrying of weapons and the wearing of kilts a penal offence. Later, Queen Victoria discovered the road north and revived the Highland games and dancing. Over time, the dance moved from male to a now 95 percent female performance.

Four standard dances remain: the Sword Dance, the Seann Triubhas, the Highland Fling, and the Reel of Tulloch.

The Highland Sword Dance is performed to the tune *Ghillie Callum*. Legend says that a Scottish prince named Malcolm Canmore crossed his sword over the sword of a defeated enemy and danced over the blades in triumph. Canmore was the son of King Duncan of Scotland whom Macbeth, the Earl of Moray, defeated and killed in the year 1040 to take the crown of Scotland. This is the same Macbeth of the Shakespeare play. It is said that Malcolm crossed his sword with that of the slain Macbeth and danced in triumph.

A male Scottish dancer's attire would not be complete without a kilt, a tartan cloth about two yards in width and four to six yards in length, overlapping in the front of the body and held together by a belt, with the length of the kilt not to pass below the middle of the knee. In ancient times the kilt was designed for the Scottish climate — warm and able to dry quickly without the discomfort of wet trousers.

The kilt was the pride of Scottish fighting men and today is the national dress of Scotland.

Dance Videos

Corryvrechan Scottish Dance Team at Kilkenny Castle: Accessed March 8, 2015, https://www.youtube.com/watch?v=G1CMN-PTYWw
Scottish Dancing at Halkirk Highland Games: Accessed March 8, 2015, https://www.youtube.com/watch?v=mCibA4BD20s
Scottish Sword Dance: Accessed February 14, 2015, http://www.youtube.com/watch?v=bZCT8H-Hpbc&feature=related

Music and Dance Trivia

Who is Donovan?
This Scottish singer and songwriter's career began in 1965 with his first single *Catch the Wind* which reached number four in the UK and peaked at number 23 in the US. His second single *Colours* was released later in 1965 and got to number four in the UK, but only managed to reach number 64 in the US. It wasn't until the release of *Sunshine Superman* in 1966, that Donovan made progress back into the charts with US number one and number two in the UK. *Mellow Yellow* quickly followed and reached number two slot in the US.

Who is Annie Lennox?

A solo artist and a member along with Dave Stewart of the duo *The Eurythmics*, which was formed in 1980 and has had several chart hits including *There Must Be an Angel (Playing with My Heart)*.

What 1968 US hit song included music played on a bagpipe?

Sky Pilot by Eric Burdon and the Animals. Near the end of the song, bagpipes can be heard, reportedly from a secret recording Burdon made of the Royal Scots Dragoon Guards playing *All the Bluebonnets Are Over the Border*. Rumor has it that this unapproved usage earned him a nasty letter from UK Royalty.

How much do beginner's bagpipes cost?

A kit including a hard case, instruction book, cassette, reeds, seasoning, hemp spool, stoppers, extra full-reed sets, and full-size rosewood Highland bagpipes costs about $300.

Name some famous tunes written for bagpipes.

Sword Dance, Corriechoillie's Welcome March, The Sweet Maid of Glendaruel, The High Road to Linton, Tail Toddle, Blue Bells of Scotland, Robin Adair, The Barren Rocks of Aden, Forty-Second Highlanders, Scotland the Brave, Highland Laddie, My Love She's But a Lassie Yet, Happy We've Been A' Thegither, The Green Hills of Tyroll, March Teribus, Earl of Mansfield's March, Corn Riggs, My Home, Rowan Tree, The Pride of Scotland. Pibroch Donald Dundee, The Invercauld March, Monymusk, The Kilt is My Delight, and *The Piper O'Drummond*.

How does a bagpipe produce sound?

The bagpipe is a wind instrument with a number of pipes and a bag. The melody pipe has finger holes that are played to produce the tune and three other pipes called drones have bass and tenor pitches. The piper puffs air into a blowpipe that fills the bag. The bag is made of animal skin and is held by the player between the side of the chest and the arm. Squeezing the bab provides air pressure to make the reeds vibrate in the chanter and drones, producing one melody and three harmonies with the one instrument.

Did other ancient countries have bagpipe players?

Some claim that the first bagpipe was made in Sumeria or China in about 5,000 BC but this has never been proven.

What is the bagpipe's connection to Egypt?
The oldest references to bagpipes appear in Alexandria, Egypt, in about 100 BC. The bagpipe may have traveled west through Europe along with spreading populations and the development of individual cultures. Both Roman and Greek writings mention bagpipes in about 100 AD. Bagpipes were known over most of Europe by about the ninth century.

What are the most popular bagpipe songs played at funerals?
Amazing Grace and *Taps*.

Why are bagpipes played at funerals?
In traditional Celtic cultures bagpipes were an important part of a traditional funeral.

Food

The native foods of Scotland include oats, fish, dairy products, local herbs, and root vegetables, plus seafood including mussels, scallops, shrimp, lobster, crabs, and many varieties of fish. Fruit includes raspberries, strawberries, tayberries, and brambles — what Americans call blackberries. Vegetables include potatoes, carrots, turnips, cabbages, and cauliflower. Lamb, game birds, and ostrich are raised as livestock.

No mention of Scottish foods would be complete without Scotch — a whiskey brewed in the country since at least 1494. By international law, no whiskey can be called Scotch unless it is brewed in Scotland. Known as the "water of life," legend says that whiskey brewing began in the late twelfth century in monasteries where it was mostly used for medicinal purposes such as relief of colic, palsy, and smallpox. Today Scotch whiskey is sold in over 200 countries around the world.

Recipe

Broken Biscuits. In the past, Scottish grocers sold loose biscuits and the broken biscuits were sold at a discount. Households also used up all food stuffs, for example leftover cake would become a new dessert. Serves 10.
Ingredients.
1 pound sweetened chocolate

1 pound butter or margarine
1 pound broken biscuits
½ pound roasted mixed nuts
1 teaspoon vanilla.

Preparation. Melt and stir the butter and chocolate together. Mix in the broken biscuits, vanilla, and nuts. Pour into a 10" by 15" baking pan lined with parchment paper. Smooth the top and leave until the mixture sets. Cut into fingers and serve.

Food Trivia

What are oatcakes?
Oatcakes were first produced in the fourteenth century by Scottish soldiers who would carry a sack of oatmeal. They would moisten and heat the oatmeal on a metal plate over a fire when they were hungry. Today, these cakes are eaten with soups or with cheese and chutney.

What is *haggis*?
Scotland's national dish, a pudding containing sheep's heart, liver, and lungs, minced with onion, oatmeal, suet, spices, and salt, and traditionally encased in the sheep's stomach. It is served with neeps and tatties (turnips and potatos), particularly when served as part of a Burns supper.

What is *tablet*?
A medium-hard and sugary sweet made from sugar, condensed milk, butter, and vanilla extract, boiled to soft-ball stage, and then allowed to crystallize. It dates back to the early eighteenth century.

True or false: Scottish salmon is sold in 55 countries around the world.
True.

What is meant by a full Scottish breakfast?
A link sausage, bacon, eggs, *tattie scone* (potato scone), fried mushrooms, grilled tomatoes, baked beans, buttered toast, white pudding, and black pudding.

What is porridge?
A traditional breakfast food, oatmeal cooked with water and a touch of salt. It is stirred with a wooden spurtle, which prevents the porridge from congealing, and served hot in a bowl.

What are kippers?
Cold smoked herring served for breakfast.

How are kippers prepared?
They are split in butterfly fashion, from tail to head, soaked in brine, and then smoked over smoldering woodchips.

Does Scotland produce cheese?
Yes, the country has over two dozen cheesemakers, ranging from large, industrial cheddar creameries to a handful of small artisans.

What traditional wild game is eaten in Scotland?
Pheasant, grouse, partridge, pigeon, hare, and rabbit.

Customs

Weddings

For three weeks before the wedding, banns were announced in church stating a couples' intent to marry to ensure that no one objected to the wedding. This practice began in medieval times and was eliminated at the beginning of the twenty-first century.

A shower of presents is a party hosted by the mother of the bride one week before the wedding. Guests bring gifts of household items for the couple's new home. Tea and cake are served to the guests.

In ancient times the bridegroom was creeled by carrying a basket (called a creel) of rocks on his back from one end of the village to the other until the bride-to-be kissed him.

Bagpipers walk ahead of the wedding party to lead them from the church to the reception where the couple lead the congregation in a reel, the first dance of the evening.

After the reception the wedding guests follow the couple to their new home where the groom lifts the bride's feet over the threshold.

Traditionally, after priests bless the home and the wedding bed, the guests leave the couple in their new home.

Children

Hanselling is a Scottish tradition in which a newborn baby is given a silver coin to bring good luck. According to legend, if the baby grasps the coin with an iron fist, that suggests he or she would grow up to be a miser, and if the coin is dropped quickly, you've got a shopaholic on your hands.

The *Howdie* is a "handy woman" who would come around when the baby was due to enact certain superstitious rituals during labor to ensure a safe delivery. Any knots, belts, or ties in the mother's clothing would be untied, onlookers would be instructed not to sit with crossed legs or arms, and all doors and windows would be unlocked, to help the baby find its way into the world. To insure the baby's soul remained free, all mirrors would be covered up and all bottles left opened. Then a potion made of rowan berries to repel fairies would be given to the mother.

After the baby was born, the Howdie would put whiskey, butter, and salt in its mouth to ward off evil spirits. All the women present would eat three spoonsful of oatmeal to fortify the baby and bring it luck.

Holidays

January 1. New Year's Day
First Monday in February. Winter Holiday
Variable date. Good Friday
Variable date. Easter
Variable date. Easter Monday
First Monday in May. Labor Day
May 25. Victoria Day
Last Monday in September. Autumn Holiday
December 25. Christmas
December 26. Boxing Day
December 31. New Year's Eve

Customs Trivia

What do men do at a child's baptism?
They raise a glass of whiskey in a toast.

What creature is bad luck at a funeral?
A black cat in any room where a wake is taking place.

What does it mean when cows lay down in the field?
Superstition says rain is coming.

Seeing what event brings bad luck on your wedding day?
A funeral procession.

Seeing what animals brings bad luck on your wedding day?
A pig.

What happens if you cut a young baby's nails with scissors?
He or she will be dishonest in later life.

What is a first footer?
The first footer is the first person to enter the home for the New Year. They should bring a lump of coal to symbolically bring heat to the house, plus a bottle of whisky and something to eat to signify plenty of food and drink in the coming year.

What happens if you cross two knifes on a table?
You will have bad luck.

What is the Curse of Scotland?
The nine of diamonds in a deck of cards because it refers to the theft of diamonds from Mary Queen of Scots.

What song is played at Scottish weddings?
The Highland Wedding.

More Resources

DVDs

Passport to England, Ireland and Scotland, DVD, Travel Channel, 2004.
Visions of Scotland, DVD, Acorn Media, 2007.

Scotland Highlands, DVD, BFS Entertainment, 2012
History of Scotland: Castles and Clans, DVD, BFS Entertainment, 2009
Scotland Revealed, DVD, BFS Entertainment, 2010

Books

Campbell, K. *United Kingdom in Pictures* (Lerner Publications, 2004).
Humphreys, R. *The Rough Guide to Scotland* (Rough Guides, 2011).
Wilson, N. *Scotland Country Travel Guide* (Lonely Planet, 2011).

Websites

Visit Scotland: Accessed December 29, 2015, www.visitscotland.com/
Scotland: Accessed March 24, 2016, http://www.scotland.org/us/
Welcome to gov.uk: Accessed December 29, 2015. www.direct.gov.uk/

Photos

Scotland Photo Gallery: Accessed December 29, 2015,
    http://www.scotland.com/photos/
Scotland Photos: Accessed December 29, 2015,
    http://www.trekearth.com/gallery/Europe/United_Kingdom/Scotland/
Scotland Photos: Accessed December 29, 2015,
    http://travel.nationalgeographic.com/travel/countries/scotland-
    photos/#/eilean-donan-castle_9064_600x450.jpg
The sixty-four most stunning pictures of Scotland ever: Accessed
    December 29, 2015,
    http://www.scotlandnow.dailyrecord.co.uk/lifestyle/heritage/64-
    most-stunning-pictures-scotland-3709630

References

Cairngorms National Park overview: Accessed December 29, 2015,
    http://www.visitscotland.com/about/nature-geography/national-parks/cairngorms
Coloring picture of Map of Scotland: Accessed December 29, 2015, http://www.coloring-
    pictures.net/drawings/Scotland/Map-of-Scotland.php
Facts About Scotland: Accessed December 29, 2015, http://www.woodlands-
    junior.kent.sch.uk/customs/questions/britain/scotland.htm
Forth Bridge: Accessed December 29, 2015, https://en.wikipedia.org/wiki/Forth_Bridge

Geography and Map of the United Kingdom: Accessed December 29, 2015,
  http://geography.about.com/library/cia/blcuk.htm
James Monroe Fast Facts: Accessed December 29, 2015,
  http://americanhistory.about.com/od/jamesmonroe/a/ff_j_monroe.htm
James Stewart: Accessed December 29, 2015, www.imdb.com/name/nm0000071/bio
Johnny Cash's Celtic Ancestry: Accessed December 29, 2015, www.johnnycash.com/
Legend of the Sword Dance: Accessed December 29, 2015,
  http://www.sohda.org.uk/article_legend_of_the_sword_dance_sohda_article.htm
Maps of Scotland: 1998-2015. Accessed December 29, 2015,
  http://www.coloring.ws/scotland.htm
Scotland Native Animals: Accessed June 29, 2012, http://www.scotland-
  placestovisit.com/twv//categories/Native-Animals/
Scottish Children's Games: Accessed December 29, 2015,
  http://www.ehow.com/list_6180471_scottish-children_s-
  games.html#ixzz1zEeROjDS
Scottish Food and Drink: Accessed December 29, 2015,
  http://www.scotland.org/experience-scotland/scottish-food-and-drink/
Scottish highland dancing: Accessed December 29, 2015,
  https://en.wikipedia.org/wiki/Scottish_highland_dance
Scottish History: Accessed December 29, 2015, http://www.scotland.org/about-
  scotland/scottish-history/
Scottish Pets: Accessed December 29, 2015,
  http://www.heartoscotland.com/Categories/ScottishPets.htm
The Authentic History of the Kilt: Accessed December 29, 2015, http://www.scottish-
  history.com/kilt.shtml
The Concise History of the Bagpipe: Accessed December 29, 2015,
  http://www.bagpipehistory.info/scotland.shtml
The Curse of Scotland: Accessed December 29, 2015,
  http://www.bbc.co.uk/scotland/history/the_curse_of_scotland.shtml
The History and Words of Auld Lang Syne: Accessed December 29, 2015,
  http://www.scotland.org/features/the-history-and-words-of-auld-lang-syne/
The Whisky Success Story: Accessed December 29, 2015,
  http://www.whisky.com/history.html
VisitScotland Highlights Celebrities with Scottish Roots: Accessed December 29, 2015,
  http://www.holyroodpr.co.uk/visitscotland_highlights_celebrities_with_scottish_roo
  ts/#sthash.D6Ef3HKv.dpuf
Washington Irving Biography: Accessed December 29, 2015,
  www.biography.com/people/washington-irving-9350087

SWEDEN

Basics

Geography

Sweden is located in Northern Europe on the Scandinavian Peninsula. It is bordered by Norway to the west and Finland to the east as well as the Baltic Sea and the Gulf of Bothnia. Sweden has three main rivers which all flow into the Gulf of Bothnia: the Ume, the Torne, and the Angerman rivers. The third largest lake in Europe, Vanern, is located in the southwestern part of the country.

Parts of Sweden are located above the Arctic Circle, thus residents there experience long and very cold winters. Because of its northern latitude, much of Sweden stays dark for longer periods during the winter and light for more hours in the summer than more southerly countries.

Language

The official language is Swedish but the country also has five additional official languages which are Finnish, Yiddish, Sami, Meänkieli, and Romani. Children are taught English in elementary schools.

History

As in much of Europe, Sweden's history began with prehistoric hunting camps. In the seventh and eighth centuries Sweden was known for its trade. In the ninth century the Vikings raided the region and much of Europe and founded the first kingdom of Russia.

Denmark's Queen Margaret created the Kalmar Union in 1397 which included Sweden, Finland, Norway, and Denmark. In the fifteenth century this union dissolved with Sweden gaining its independence in 1523.

During the seventh century Sweden and Finland, which was then a part of Sweden, fought and won several wars against Denmark, Russia, and Poland. By 658 Sweden controlled many areas including several provinces in Denmark, but this was short-lived as Russia, Saxony-Poland, and Denmark-Norway attacked Sweden in 700, ending Sweden's period as a powerful country.

Sweden was forced to cede Finland to Russia in 1809. In 1813 Sweden fought against Napoleon and shortly thereafter the Congress of Vienna created a merger between Sweden and Norway, a dual monarchy, which was peacefully dissolved in 1905.

During the 1800s Sweden's decision to shift its economy to private agriculture was a failure and between 1850 and 1890 about a million Swedes moved to the US. Sweden remained neutral in World War I and produced essential products including steel, ball bearings, and matches. After the war, the country's economy improved and social welfare policies were developed. Sweden joined the European Union in 1995.

Map and Flag

Sweden Map: Accessed March 21, 2015,
   http://www.supercoloring.com/pages/sweden-map
The Flag of Sweden: Accessed March 21, 2015,
   http://www.enchantedlearning.com/europe/sweden/flag/

Travel

Distance

From New York, NY, to Stockholm is 3,937 miles. Flight time is 8 hours 22 minutes.

From Chicago, IL, to Stockholm is 4,287 miles. Flight time is 9 hours 4 minutes.

From Dallas, TX, to Stockholm is 5,084 miles. Flight time is 10 hours 40 minutes.

From Seattle, WA, to Stockholm is 4,731 miles. Flight time is 9 hours 58 minutes.

Hotels

Gorvalns Slott. Located in Gorvalnsvagen, Jarfalla, near the beach. It allows pets and has an on-site restaurant and bar.

Icehotel. Located in Jukkasjärv, it is the world's largest hotel made of ice and snow. The 5,500 square meter complex includes an Icechurch and an Icebar. Constructed anew every November and December, it melts in April and May. It features snow rooms, ice rooms, and art suites. Guests may book a wide range of snowmobile excursions such as Arctic Trail which goes through the wilderness trails of Swedish Lapland's aboriginal Sami people, whose life is integrally tied to reindeer migration. Other tour options are fishing for char, trout, and grayling, sauna and dinner programs, ice driving, moose watching, ice sculpting, Northern Lights viewing, and dog sled safaris.

Lydmar Hotel. Located in Stockholm overlooking the Royal Palace, Parliament, harbor, and the back side of the Strand.

Stora Hotellet Umea. Located in Umea next to the town hall. It has a restaurant and bar and features free breakfast for guests.

Upper House. Located in Gothenburg, it features luxury beds, a heated glass-bottomed swimming pool, a spa, and free breakfast.

Landmarks

Gothenburg. The capital of West Sweden features canals and Sweden's largest botanical garden with over 16,000 species.

Kosterhavet. Sweden's first marine national park, near fishing villages surrounded by plants and flowers along the beaches and rocky islands. Tourists can enjoy seal safaris, swimming, and diving.

Museum Gustavianum. Located in Uppsala, it features Uppsala University memorabilia and information about Viking graves.

Stockholm Archipelago. An area of more than 30,000 islands accessible by boat all year round. Tourist trips range from one hour to overnight stays and many include meals.

Tylosand Strand. Located in Halmstad, it features miles of beautiful beaches for swimming, kite surfing, and sunset watching.

Vasa Museum. Located in Stockholm, it features the Vasa, a ship built in 1628 which sank in the harbor on her maiden voyage and was salvaged in 1961 after lying on the bottom of the harbor for 333 years. The museum also houses many artifacts.

Travel Trivia

What is the official name of Sweden
The Kingdom of Sweden.

True or false: Sweden is one of the smallest counties in Europe.
False: In land size Sweden is the fourth largest in Europe.

What is the capitol of Sweden?
Stockholm.

True or false: Sweden has many national parks.
True. Forests cover more than 60 percent of Sweden and there are also around 100,000 lakes and over 30,000 islands. Sweden's public access laws allows the public to fully access these areas.

True or false: The Swedish Vikings of the eighth through tenth centuries were a fearsome group, highly skilled at warfare, and they invaded and settled throughout Northern and Eastern Europe.
True. During the seventh century Sweden again emerged as a great power in Europe with the Swedish Empire gaining territories in Eastern Europe.

True or false: Sweden has remain neutral in all wars since 1814, including World Wars I and II.
True.

True or false: Military service is mandated in Sweden.
True. All Swedes over 19 year of age must complete up to 15 months of military service.

Name a manufacturing or technology company founded in Sweden.
Ericsson, Volvo, Saab, IKEA, and Electrolux.

True or false: Sweden was the first country to grant suffrage for married women.
True, in 1862.

True or false: Sweden has the most personal computers per person.
True. One for every two people.

What astronomy tool was invented in Sweden?
The astronomical lens.

What form of power does Sweden have more of per capita than anywhere else?
Nuclear power.

True or false: Sweden has the highest number of women lawmakers in the world.
True. Forty-seven percent of the parliament are women.

True or false: In Sweden everyone, even graduate students, get five weeks of paid vacation per year.
True.

True or false: Right turn on red is allowed on all Swedish streets.
False. It is prohibited everywhere.

Is there tuition at Swedish universities?
No. Students pay only a student union membership fee.

How long does the average Swede spend in formal education?
Until age 25.

True or false: You may camp anywhere in Sweden except on military or private property.
True.

True or false: In Sweden you can receive sick leave while on vacation.
True.

How much is the income tax in Sweden?
Between 50 and 70 percent of your income.

America's Roots

Who is Taylor Swift?
A popular singer who grew up in Pennsylvania. She has Swedish ancestors.

Who is George W. Bush?
The forty-third US president. He has Swedish ancestors.

Who was Abraham Lincoln?
The sixteenth US president. He had Swedish ancestors.

Who is George H. W. Bush?
The forty-first US president. He was of Swedish descent.

Who is Buzz Aldrin?
An astronaut and the second person to walk on the surface of the moon. He has Swedish ancestors.

Who was Charles Lindbergh?
An aviator who was the first to fly solo across the Atlantic Ocean. His father came to the US from Sweden as an infant.

Who was Ray Bradbury?
An author of many books including *Fahrenheit 451*. He was born in Illinois and his mother was from Sweden.

Who was Mamie Eisenhower?
First lady to the thirty-fourth US President Dwight D. Eisenhower. Her maternal grandparents were from Sweden.

Who is Gretchen Carlson?
A journalist and Fox News anchor. Born in Minnesota, she is of Swedish descent.

Who was Carl Sandburg?
Born in Illinois, he was an author and poet who won three Pulitzer Prizes. Both his parents were of Swedish descent.

Who is Tipper Gore?
She was born in Washington DC, was married to the forty-fifth US vice president Al Gore, and is of Swedish ancestry.

Who is Susan Lucci?
An actress well-known for her Emmy-winning role on the TV soap opera *All My Children*. She was born in New York and her mother is of Swedish ancestry.

Who is Robert Englund?
An actor and the star of the horror movie series *Nightmare on Elm Street*. He was born in California, is of Swedish ancestry, and speaks fluent Swedish.

Who was Ozzie Nelson?
An actor, band leader, and producer of the TV show *Ozzie and Harriet*. His paternal grandparents were from Sweden.

Sports and Games

Sports

The most popular sport in Sweden is football, which Americans call soccer, followed by ice hockey. There are junior ice hockey teams throughout the country and almost every Swedish boy has played ice hockey.

Bandy is a game created in Sweden in 1894 which today is played in Russia, the Netherlands, and Hungary. The game has 11 players on each team and three substitute players. It is played on an ice-covered field about the size of a US football field. The ball is made with a cork center and hit with a wooden club similar to but smaller than a hockey stick. The game has two 45 minute sessions and you win by gaining the most goals during this time period.

Other athletics, including the steeplechase, high jump, and javelin, are very popular in the country. Children begin playing in local teams at age 11 and pick a specialization within their sport at age 15.

Orienteering in Sweden is not only about finding your way with a map and a compass, but also how quickly you reach each check point on the course. Contestants' cards are stamped to prove when they reached each checkpoint. Courses may take players through swamps and over rocky fields. The sport is a popular family activity and annually attracts more than 100,000 participants.

Other popular Swedish sports include swimming with most cities having a public pool, gymnastics, martial arts, and horseback riding.

Sports Trivia

What is Gothenborg?
The location of the Gothenburg Horse Show, one of the world's most famous series of Grand Prix horse jumping competitions.

What is the Swedish Budo Association?
The umbrella organization for martial arts in Sweden which includes the Swedish Judo Association and the Swedish Karate Association.

When was the first international *bandy* league formed?
In 1902 in Sweden.

Who is Phil Mickelson?
An American professional golfer of Swedish descent.

Who is Bob Burnquist?
An American professional skateboarder of Swedish descent.

What is the O-ringen?
One of the largest orienteering competitions in Sweden.

What is the DN-Galen?
An athletics competition held every July in Sweden which is part of the European Grand Prix Tour.

What Swedish organization teaches the nation's children to swim?
The Swedish Life Saving Association.

How many clubs belong to the Swedish Gymnastic Federation?
More than 68.

Game

Kubb. A popular Swedish outdoor game, modified for residents' indoor use.

Number of players. Ten, in two teams of five players each.

Materials. To construct 10 kubbs, the king, six batons, and four stakes, you will need a 6' long 4x4, 6' of 1.5"-2" dowel, 4' of ¾" dowel, and 30' of brightly colored masking tape.

To make the king, cut 12" off the 4x4. Then make two 45-degree cuts into the sides. To make the kubbs, note that the size of a kubb is 2¾" x 2¾" x 5⅞" so trim ¾" off two sides of the remaining 4x4, then cut the 4x4 into ten 5⅞" pieces. To make the six batons and four stakes, cut the dowels into ten 12" lengths.

Mark off a 5' x 2' playing area on the floor with bright colored tape.

To play. Place the king in the center of the playing area. Place five kubbs, one at either end, one in the middle, and the remaining two equidistant between the end and middle kubbs.

Each team goes to their end of the playing area.

Batons must always be thrown vertically and underarm. To decide which team goes first, one person from each team throws a baton as close to the king as possible without hitting it. The team with the stick closest to the king starts.

For the first turn only, four batons are thrown from behind the home baseline at the opponent's baseline kubbs. Players collect any kubbs toppled during the opponents' turn. These kubbs are then thrown from the baseline into the opponents' half of the court.

If a kubb comes to rest outside the opponent's half of the court, players have one more chance to get it right by retrieving it and throwing it again. If a kubb fails to land in the required part of the opponents' area the second time, then the opponents can place it anywhere they like on their side of the court, although it must be at least one stick length away from their king. In doing so, players are usually aiming to make the kubbs land just beyond the middle line because the nearer the kubbs are, the easier they are to topple in the next phase of the turn.

If there are any batons left over once all the kubbs on the opponents' side have been toppled, then players may aim at the king. When throwing at the king, players must throw from behind the baseline.

When the team has thrown its six batons without knocking over the king, the turn passes back to the first team, and the entire procedure is repeated.

Winner. If the king is knocked over by a thrown kubb or by a baton before all the kubbs on the opponent's side have been toppled, then the team that knocked it over loses and their opponents have won. Otherwise, the game is won by the team that first topples all the kubbs on the opponents' half of the court and then topples the king from behind the baseline.

ICHI benefits. Physical balance, mobility of joints, muscle tone, control of voluntary movement, mental functions of language, speech, and articulation.

Music and Dance

Music

Folk music, *folkmusik* in Swedish, is alive and well throughout the country in many music and dance organizations.

The traditional instruments are the fiddle and the accordion, but some folk musicians also play the clarinet, the recorder, a single reed bagpipe, the *salgflojt* which is an overtone flute made of willow, and the *spelpipa* which is a traditional whistle. A *nyckelharpa* is a fiddle unique to Sweden

The most common kind of accordion is the five-row button *femradigt dragspel* which has the same note on push and pull. Piano accordions called *pianodragspel* are also common.

Accordions or melodeons with different notes on push and pull are called *durspel*. The most common kinds are two-row or *tvaradigt* and one-row or *enradigt* accordions.

Folk music festivals are held throughout Sweden, ranging from a small gathering called a *spelmansstamma* meaning *musicians meeting* which is held once a year to events attended by thousands of people and held over several days, usually in the summer months. In the midst of these events many people play together in small informal groups in what is called *buskspel* meaning playing in the bushes. At most meetings there is also a *visstuga*, a singing session, held in a house.

Music Videos

Music of Sweden: Accessed April 2, 2015,
    https://www.youtube.com/watch?v=JeE5DP8dyWU
Swedish Baroque: Accessed April 2, 2015,
    https://www.youtube.com/watch?v=SQJm63jgJeE
Swedish Folk Music Live: Accessed April 2, 2015,
    https://www.youtube.com/watch?v=k9j212da4CU

Swedish folk song: Accessed April 2, 2015,
  https://www.youtube.com/watch?v=wA8DfZZAQxc
Swedish Folk Song. Red Socks Band: Accessed April 2, 2015,
  https://www.youtube.com/watch?v=BhBew_VQKtM

Dance

All dance begins with a rhythmic tune and in Swedish music the most popular is the *polska*, a dance tune played in 3/4 time but in the same style as the waltz. About 75 percent of all the dance tunes played by Swedish folk musicians are in polska rhythm.

Other common dances are waltzes, polkas, and mazurkas. There are walking and marching tunes and traditional wedding marches.

How is polska different from a waltz? Polskas are played at a slower pace and with different stress on the beats. A waltz has three beats per measure, clapped out as *bom-bip-bip*. A polska would clap out as *bom-bip-bom*.

The *polska* has been part of the country's history since the late 1500s. There are several forms including the *langpolska* which is a serpentine or line dance believed to have originated in the Middle Ages.

The polska is mostly a couples dance now. During the Middle Ages European ring dances often concluded with a swinging of partners which became a dance separate from the rest of the dance. Varieties today include *Svangpolska* (swinging or wheeling polska), Korpolska (trotting polska), *Bondpolska* (farmer's polska), *Delsbopolska* (Devil's polska), and *Svingedans* (swinging dance).

Dance Videos

Swedish Folk Dance: Accessed April 2, 2015,
  https://www.youtube.com/watch?v=1reedKeVdmY
Swedish Folk Dance: Accessed April 2, 2015,
  https://www.youtube.com/watch?v=k9j212da4CU
Swedish Traditional Dance: Accessed April 2, 2015,
  https://www.youtube.com/watch?v=QwZVbqY4ivs
Swedish Traditional Dance: Accessed April 2, 2015,
  https://www.youtube.com/watch?v=xI3rUtzxLRQ

Swedish Traditional Folk Dance: Hambo and Vava Vadmal: Accessed
April 2, 2015, https://www.youtube.com/watch?v=3plkx_z6Xn4

Music and Dance Trivia

What is a *Nacken*?
A water spirit who lives in Swedish streams and plays the fiddle.

What can a *Nacken* do?
According to folklore he can teach you to play the fiddle so well that
your listeners will not be able to stop their feet from tapping.

Who is Grace Slick?
A singer of Swedish descent who, with her band *Jefferson Airplane*
wrote and performed hit songs such as *White Rabbit* and *Volunteers*.

Who is Kris Kristofferson?
A musician, actor, songwriter, and film score composer of Swedish
descent.

Who is Todd Rundgren?
A musician, recording engineer, songwriter, and music producer of
Swedish descent.

Who was *ABBA*?
ABBA was a Swedish band formed in Stockholm in 1972 which had
worldwide hits from 1975 to 1982.

How did *ABBA* make history in 1974?
By winning the Eurovision Song Contest 1974 at the Dome in Brighton,
UK, giving Sweden its first triumph in the history of the contest.

What is Europe?
A Swedish heavy metal/hard rock formed in 1979.

Who is Anne Sofie von Otter?
A well-known Swedish mezzo-soprano opera singer.

Who was Christina Nilsson, Countess de Casa Miranda?
A Swedish operatic soprano who became a member of the Royal
Swedish Academy of Music in 1869.

Food

Sweden's food history began with the Vikings who prepared for long, cold winters by preserving meat, fish, fruits, and vegetables. They were the first to develop a method for preserving foods. In preparation for long voyages, foods were salted, dehydrated, and cured. While refrigeration and freezing has eliminated the need for these preserving methods, Swedes continue to salt, dehydrate, and cure many of their foods, particularly fish.

From 800 to 1050 AD, the Vikings raided lands throughout Europe and as far south as the Mediterranean Sea. They returned to Sweden with tea from England, French sauces and soups, and honey cakes from Germany which became part of the Swedish diet. Many Swedes still make soup as a way to use leftover food.

The Swedes prefer European foods, and even restaurants in Sweden tend to serve more foreign dishes. However, historians believe it was the Swedes who introduced fruit soups, smoked meats, cream sauces, and herring to early Russians.

Swedish *smorgasbord* is a style of home cooking in which a number of small hot and cold dishes are served buffet-style. The literal meaning of the word is bread and butter table. The term smorgasbord has become world famous, representing a collection of various foods presented all at once.

Foods served in a traditional smorgasbord are herring, smoked eel, roast beef, jellied fish, boiled potatoes, a layered potato dish containing onions and cream and topped with anchovies, and *kottbulla* which are Swedish meatballs.

Recipe

Creamy Dipping Sauce is traditionally served with fish or over vegetables. This recipe can be used with residents on regular diets, those on mechanical soft diets when used to dip bread, and as a taste for those on puréed diets.

Ingredients.
¾ cup butter
4 egg yolks, whites discarded
1½ cups cream

Lemon juice to taste.

Preparation. Melt the butter in the top of a double boiler over simmering, not boiling, water. Beat the egg yolks with the cream until stiff. Add the cream and egg mixture to the butter, beating constantly until the sauce is foamy and slightly thick. Remove from the stove and add the lemon juice to taste.

Food Trivia

What are lingonberries?
A fruit which grows wild in the forests of Sweden. Public access allows citizens to pick fruit in forests. This fruit is used to make lingonberry jam which is used to garnish food in the same way Americans use mustard and ketchup.

Can I spread lingonberry jam on bread?
Swedes consider it too sweet for bread.

What is pickled herring?
A favorite Swedish meal with a variety of flavorings from onion to mustard and garlic to dill. It is served with boiled potatoes, boiled eggs, and crisp bread.

What is crisp bread?
A hard, thin baked good that when stored properly can last a year. It is served at every meal and has been a staple in Sweden for over 500 years.

What is the traditional Swedish food on Thursdays?
Pea soup and pancakes.

Why eat pea soup on Thursday?
Folklore says the practice began because pea soup is easy to make and maids who worked only a half-day on Thursdays served it as a quick meal.

Why eat pancakes on Thursdays?
This tradition began during World War II when the Swedish Armed Forces ate pancakes topped with jam.

How do you prepare crisp bread?
You make the dough, roll it out, and hang it to dry.

What is the favorite dessert in Sweden?
Green princess cake, a yellow sponge cake filled with jam, vanilla custard, and heavy cream, and topped with a bright pink sugar rose.

What is the legend of princess cake?
Jenny Akerstrom, a teacher, made it in 1920 for the daughters of Prince Carl Bernadotte. It is served for special occasions and during the third week of September which is called Princess Cake Week.

Customs

Weddings

Swedish weddings, called *bröllop*, typically take place in a church as an afternoon ceremony. No one gives the bride away, and there is no maid of honor, best man, flower girls, bridesmaids, or groomsmen. In Sweden the couple walks down the aisle together and are joined at the altar by one best friend each. After the ceremony the couple is greeted by their family and friends who throw raw rice on the couple before going to the reception.

Traditionally a Swedish bride wore a garland of myrtle on her head as a symbol of innocence, and a folk wedding costume. Modern brides wear a white dress and tiara or veil. The bride also carries coins in her shoes and, once married, wears three wedding rings which represent engagement, marriage, and motherhood.

Forget about catching the bride's bouquet at a Swedish reception. In Sweden the lucky bride keeps her flowers. Lots of speeches from any and all guests can continue throughout the dinner.

During the party traditional Swedish wedding folk songs are performed, and at most weddings every table has a copy of the lyrics so guests can join in the singing. Tossing a drink of vodka onto the couple is also a custom.

Children

Choosing the name of a child is not completely up to the parents. The Swedish naming law enacted in 1982 was originally created to prevent non-noble families from giving their children noble names. There are also additional restrictions in the law: "First names shall not be approved if they can cause offense or can be supposed to cause discomfort for the one using it, or names which for some obvious reason are not suitable as a first name."

First names must be reported to the Swedish Tax Agency. You may have multiple first names, but if you later change your name you must keep at least one of the first names that you were originally given, and you can only change your name once. For example, if you're named John and want to change to Jack, your new first name will be Jack John, keeping the original first name. Any further changes must be made through the Swedish Patent and Registration Office.

Examples of rejected names include Metallica, Superman, Veranda, Ikea, and Elvis. However, some surprising names were permitted such as Google as a middle name and Lego as a first name.

If the parents do not select a last name, the child is given the surname of the mother. Both parents attend the childbirth and there are continuing parental education classes for mothers and fathers.

Holidays

January 1. New Year's Day
January 6. Epiphany
Variable date. Good Friday
Variable date. Easter
Variable date. Easter Monday
First Monday in May. Labor Day
Variable date. Ascension
June 6. National Day
June 19. Midsummer's Eve
October 31. All Saints' Day
November 8. Father's Day
December 25. Christmas
December 26. Boxing Day
December 31. New Year's Eve

Customs Trivia

Why does the bride carry coins in her shoes?
One silver coin in her left shoe from her father and one gold coin in her right from her mother are meant to ensure that she will never go without.

What happens if the groom leaves his wedding reception?
Tradition dictates if the groom leaves the room for any reason, then the other men at the wedding are allowed to kiss the bride! And vice versa!

What is the Swedish name for wedding songs?
Brollopgfest.

What determines who will be the leader in the marriage?
The custom is that whoever shouts "I do!" the loudest will rule the marriage.

What time of the year is most common for weddings?
Summer, to avoid the harsh weather of other seasons.

True or false: You may not breastfeed in public in Sweden.
False: Breastfeeding can be done in public spaces.

True or false: Infants sleep in the same bed as their parents.
True. Parent-child co-sleeping is the norm.

How long is maternity leave in Sweden?
It starts two months before birth and lasts 15 months.

Why is maternity leave so long?
To allow mothers a generous time for breastfeeding.

True or false: Childcare is 100 percent paid by the parents.
False: Childcare is publicly funded, open to all children, and used by the majority of families.

More Resources

DVDs

Cities of the World, Stockholm, Sweden, DVD, TravelVideoStore.com, 2009.

Cities of the World, Sweden, DVD, TravelVideoStore.com, 2011.
Esovision Husky Safari Sweden, DVD, Global Television, 2012
On Tour...Call of the Wild Life with the Huskies Sweden, DVD, Global Television, 2012.
Return to Sweden, DVD, TravelVideoStore.com, 2010.

Books

Carr, L. and C. Robinowitz. *Modern-Day Vikings: A Pracical Guide to Interacting with the Swedes* (Intercultural Press, 2001).
DeWitt, C. Sweden — *Culture Smart!: the essential guide to customs & culture* (Kuperard, 2012).
DK Publishing. *DK Eyewitness Travel Guide: Sweden* (DK Publishing, 2013).
Ohlsen, B., A. Kaminski, and K. Lundergren. *Lonely Planet Sweden* (Lonely Planet, 2012).
Proctor, J. and N. Roland. *The Rough Guide to Sweden* (Rough Guides, 2012).

Websites

Flag of Sweden: Accessed March 21, 2015, http://www.flags.net/SWDN.htm
Government Offices of Sweden: Accessed March 21, 2015, ttp://www.government.se/
Map of Sweden: Accessed March 21, 2015, http://www.sverigeturism.se/smorgasbord/smorgasbord/service/sweden-map.html
Sweden's official website for tourism and travel information: Accessed March 21, 2015, http://www.visitsweden.com/sweden-us/
US Department of State. Sweden: Accessed March 21, 2015, http://travel.state.gov/content/passports/english/country/sweden.html

Photos

Image Bank. Sweden: Accessed March 21, 2015, http://www.tripadvisor.com/LocationPhotos-g189806-w2-Sweden.html

Photos of Sweden: Accessed March 21, 2015,
   http://www.tripadvisor.com/LocationPhotos-g189806-w2-
   Sweden.html
Planetware. Sweden. 2015. Accessed March 21, 2015,
   http://www.planetware.com/pictures/sweden-s.htm
Sweden: Accessed March 21, 2015,
   http://travel.nationalgeographic.com/travel/countries/sweden-guide/
Sweden Photo Gallary: Accessed March 21, 2015,
   http://goscandinavia.about.com/od/photogalleries/ig/Sweden-Photo-
   Gallery/

References

50+ Famous People of Swedish Descent: Accessed March 21, 2015,
   http://www.ranker.com/list/famous-people-of-swedish-descent/celebrity-
   lists?format=SLIDESHOW&page=36
Amusing Facts about Sweden: Accessed March 17, 2015,
   http://cva.stanford.edu/people/davidbbs/swedish_facts.html
Best Luxury Hotels in Sweden: Accessed March 16, 2015,
   http://www.tripadvisor.com/TravelersChoice-Hotels-cLuxury-g189806
Countries with Fascinating Naming Laws: Accessed March 21, 2015,
   http://mentalfloss.com/article/25034/8-countries-fascinating-baby-naming-laws
Country Facts. Sweden: Accessed March 17, 2015,
   http://www.sciencekids.co.nz/sciencefacts/countries/sweden.html
Famous Opera Singers from Sweden: Accessed March 21, 2015,
   http://www.ranker.com/list/famous-opera-singers-from-sweden/reference?page=2
Food by Country. Sweden: Accessed March 21, 2015,
   http://www.foodbycountry.com/Spain-to-Zimbabwe-Cumulative-
   Index/Sweden.html
Geography of Sweden: Accessed March 16, 2015,
   http://geography.about.com/od/swedenmaps/a/geography-of-sweden.htm
Historical Notes on Swedish Hambo: Accessed March 21, 2015,
   http://www.phantomranch.net/folkdanc/articles/historical_notes_hambo_tracie.htm
How to Make a Kubb Set: Accessed March 21, 2015,
   http://www.instructables.com/id/How-to-Make-a-Kubb-Set/
Interesting Facts About Sweden: Accessed March 17, 2015,
   http://www.eupedia.com/sweden/trivia.shtml
Languages of the World. Sweden: Accessed March 16, 2015,
   http://languagesoftheworld.info/geolinguistics/languages-of-sweden.html
Most Popular Sports in Sweden: Accessed March 21, 2015,
   http://www.sverigeturism.se/smorgasbord/smorgasbord/natrecspo/sports/popular.ht
   ml
Swedish Traditional Music: Accessed March 21, 2015, http://www.norbeck.nu/swedtrad/

Swedish Wedding Traditions: Customs and Culture: Accessed March 21, 2015,
http://www.yourlivingcity.com/stockholm/community/swedish-wedding-traditions-customs-culture/

Ten Best Places to Visit in Sweden: Accessed March 17, 2015,
http://www.neverstoptraveling.com/the-top-10-places-in-sweden

Ten Things to Know About Swedish Food: Accessed March 21, 2015,
https://sweden.se/culture-traditions/10-things-to-know-about-swedish-food/

The Rules of Kubb: Accessed March 21, 2015,
http://www.mastersgames.com/rules/kubb-rules.htm

Top Ten Attractions — Sweden: Accessed March 17, 2015,
http://www.tripadvisor.com/TravelersChoice-Destinations-cTop-g189806

Travel Math. Sweden: Accessed March 16, 2015,
http://www.travelmath.com/from/Seattle,+WA/to/Stockholm,+Sweden

SWITZERLAND

Basics

Geography

Switzerland is located between northern and southern Europe. The country is bordered by France and Germany to the north, Austria and Liechtenstein to the east, Italy to the south, and France again on the south and southwest. The country's area is 15,942 square miles which is slightly less than twice the size of New Jersey.

Switzerland's three main geographical regions are the Jura which is a chain of mountains, the Plateau, and the Alps. Switzerland has six per cent of Europe's fresh water. The Rhine, Rhone, and Inn rivers all have their source in Switzerland and from there flow into three seas: the North Sea, the Mediterranean, and the Black Sea.

The Rhine Falls, at 450 feet wide and 75.4 feet high, are the largest in Europe. The country also has over 1,500 lakes, including Lake Geneva, which is located near the Rhone and is the largest freshwater lake in central Europe.

Language

The country has four official languages: German, French, Italian, and Rumantsch. German is used in northern, central, and eastern Switzerland, French in western Switzerland, Italian in southern Switzerland, and Rumantsch in southeastern Switzerland.

History

Switzerland was originally inhabited by the Helvetians, or Helvetic Celts. Recorded history begins with the Roman conquest in 1 BC. The Romans remained in power through 4 AD and during this period the Roman road system was built through the cities of Geneva, Basel, and Zurich.

After the fall of the Roman Empire, the country was invaded by Germanic tribes. In 800 AD it became part of Charlemagne's empire and then was ruled by a series of Holy Roman emperors. In 1291 AD Swiss ruling families from Uri, Schwyz, and Unterwalden signed a charter to keep public peace and pledging mutual support in upholding autonomous administrative and judicial rule. The anniversary of the charter's signing is celebrated as Switzerland's National Day.

Switzerland gained independence from the Holy Roman Empire in 1499. Napoleon invaded and annexed much of the country in 1798. In 1815 the Congress of Vienna established Switzerland's status of permanent armed neutrality in international law.

The country remained neutral during World Wars I and II. Switzerland did not join the United Nations until 2002 and has never joined the European Union.

Map and Flag

Flag of Switzerland to Color: Accessed March 15, 2015,
   http://www.hellokids.com/c_1585/coloring-pages/countries-coloring-pages/maps-coloring-pages/switzerland-map

Switzerland Map Coloring Page. Accessed March 15, 2015,
   http://www.hellokids.com/c_1585/coloring-pages/countries-coloring-pages/maps-coloring-pages/switzerland-map

Travel

Distance

From New York, NY, to Berne is 3,908 miles. Flight time is 8 hours 19 minutes.

From Chicago, IL, to Berne is 4, 416 miles. Flight time is 9 hours 20 minutes.

From Dallas, TX, to Berne is 5,214 miles. Flight time is 10 hours 56 minutes.

From Seattle, WA, to Berne is 5,255 miles. Flight time is 11 hours 1 minute.

Hotels

Baur au Lac. Located in Zurich it is a 168-year-old family-owned hotel overlooking Lake Zürich which features a chocolate tasting bar.

Grand Hotel National Lucerne. Located in Lucerne, it features an indoor pool, sauna, access to a Kneipp hydrotherapy and salt lounge, and a cosmetic suite and facials.

Hotel Castell. Located in Engadine St. Moritz and features a rock water sauna designed by Tadashi Kawamata. It also offers skiing and professional childcare.

Riffelalp Resort. Located in Zermatt, it features both indoor and outdoor pools as well as a view of the Matterhorn.

Rocks Resort. Located in Laax, it features a view of the Alps and is the perfect place for snowboarding.

Landmarks

Château de Chillon. A castle overlooking Lake Geneva which was built in the thirteenth century. It has courtyards, towers, halls filled with arms, period furniture, artwork, and even a dungeon. It became famous in 1816 when Lord Byron wrote *The Prisoner of Chillon*, a poem about François Bonivard who was thrown into the dungeon for his seditious ideas. He was freed by Bernese forces in 1536.

Fondation Pierre Gianadda. Located in Martigny, this museum houses a collection of art by Picasso, Cézanne, and Van Gogh, as well as a collection of Roman vessels and classic cars from vintage Fords to Swiss Martinis.

Fraumunster. A thirteenth-century cathedral renowned for its stained-glass windows which were designed by the Russian-Jewish master Marc Chagall who created a series of five windows in the choir stalls and the rose window in the southern transept. The rose window in the northern transept was created by Augusto Giacometti in 1945.

Gletscherschlucht. Located in Grindelwald, it is a natural glacier gorge where rough waters carved a path of tunnels into cliffs veined with pink and green marble. A popular spot for canyon and bungee jumping expeditions.

Matterhorn. One of the world's most renowned and historical mountains, it is surrounded by spectacular alpine scenery and Swiss villages. The trail around the Matterhorn crosses between Italy and Switzerland. Hikers can make good use of the steel ropes mounted along the path of a very challenging hike.

Stiftsbibliothek. Located in St. Gallen, this sixteenth-century library is filled with priceless books and manuscripts handwritten by monks during the Middle Ages. During tours you can see the monks' filing system hidden in the wall panels and a 2,700-year-old mummified corpse.

Travel Trivia

What is the official name of Switzerland?
Switzerland and Confoederatio Helvetica.

What international charity was founded in Switzerland?
he International Committee of the Red Cross in Geneva in 1863.

Why is the flag of the Red Cross red and white?
It is an inverted version of the Swiss flag to symbolize where the relief organization was founded.

Where is the longest staircase in the world?
The Swiss Niesenbahn with 11,674 steps.

How many mountain peaks are in Switzerland?
208 mountains over 9,000 feet high and 24 over 13,000 feet tall.

What wearable device was invented in Switzerland?
The wristwatch in 1868.

What is the oldest watch making firm in the world?
Vacheron Constantin in Geneva was founded in 1755 and is still operating.

What is the dry wind that blows through the Alps in the winter?
Foehn, similar to the Chinook winds in North America.

What is the most famous mountain in Switzerland?
The Matterhorn which is 14,692 feet high.

How much of Switzerland is covered by mountains?
Seventy percent.

What is the highest mountain in Switzerland?
Monte Rosa, at 15,203 feet.

What is the largest glacier in Switzerland?
Aletschgletscher which is about 73.3 square miles in size.

What is the capitol of Switzerland?
Bern, which is also the fourth largest city in the country.

What is the name of the castle that inspired Lord Bryon to write *The Prisoner of Chillon*?
Montreux.

What are the natural resources of Switzerland?
Hydropower, timber, and salt.

What does the country export?
Machinery, chemicals, metals, watches, and agricultural products.

What is the currency?
The Swiss franc.

What mountain range runs through the country?
The Jura.

What is the literacy rate?
Ninety-nine percent for those over age 15.

What is the largest city?
Zurich.

America's Roots

Who was Louis Chevrolet?
Founder of Chevrolet Motor Car Company in 1911. He was born in Switzerland in 1878. He raced in the Indianapolis 500 four times with his best finish seventh place in 1919.

Who was Adolf Meyer?
A psychiatrist born in Switzerland in 1866, he advocated socialized medicine, and studied symptoms. Beginning in 1910 he chaired the department of psychiatry at Johns Hopkins Medical School.

Who was Ferdinand Hassler?
A mathematician and scientist born in 1770 in Switzerland. In 1807 he designed a plan for a coastal survey of the US which is still valid.

Who was Adolphe Bandelier?
A geologist and explorer born in 1840 in Switzerland, he studied Mexico, the American Southwest, and Bolivia.

Who was Heinrich Kruesi?
A machinist born in 1843 in Switzerland, he worked with Thomas A. Edison in the early 1870s and became general manager and chief engineer of the Edison Machine Works in Schenectady.

Who was William Lescaze?
An architect born in Switzerland in 1896, he moved to the United States in 1921 and became famous building skyscrapers.

Who was Othmar Ammann?
An engineer born in 1879 in Switzerland, he built the George Washington and other suspension bridges in New York City.

What US President has Swiss ancestors?
President Barack Obama's seventh-great grandfather on his mother's side was born in Switzerland in 1692.

Who was Martin Vosseler?
A Swiss adventurer who walked across the US from west to east to promote better use of energy.

What US city hosts an annual festival celebrating Swiss cheese?
Green County Cheese Days occurs in Monroe, Wisconsin.

What American president helped feed the hungry?
In 1927 Herbert Hoover quickly raised 15 million dollars for supplies for victims of a Mississippi River flood, including establishing tent cities for 600,000 homeless. His family roots have been traced to twelfth-century Switzerland.

What American town hosts an annual Swiss wine festival?
Vevay, Indiana.

Who was Mary Katherine Campbell?
The only Miss America winner to hold the title twice, in 1922 and 1923. Her mother was of partial Swiss ancestry.

Who is Chesley Sullenberger?
The American airline transport pilot who successfully carried out the emergency ditching of US Airways Flight 1549 in the Hudson River, saving the lives of the 155 people on the aircraft. His ancestors are Swiss.

Who was J. Edgar Hoover?
The first Director of the US Federal Bureau of Investigation (FBI). He was of Swiss ancestry.

Sports and Games

Sports

Soccer, called football in Switzerland (there is no American-style football in the country), is the most popular sport. There are two professional national soccer teams and several regional teams as well as many amateur soccer teams throughout the country. In addition, there are over 14,000 registered women soccer players, but most of the country's attention is focused on male players. Other popular professional team sports are ice hockey whose professional teams include players from the US, Canada, and Sweden, volleyball which is the most popular among women, basketball, and handball.

As individual sports the Swiss enjoy jogging, mid-and long-distance running, and Nordic walking. Running races are held in 22 Swiss cities with competitions for men, women, and children. Race length can be 1 mile, 5 miles, or 10 miles. Traditional armed races for men required the participants to run wearing a Swiss Army uniform and carrying an army backpack and a rifle.

Located in the mountains, most Swiss towns have an ice rink which is popular with school children and adults for ice skating and ice hockey. Downhill skiing and snowboarding are usually part of every Swiss family vacation.

Swimming lessons are required in Swiss schools and many schools have indoor pools. There are also outdoor pools throughout the country.

Other warm-weather sports include biking, roller-blade skating, hiking, climbing, horseback riding, golfing, sailing, windsurfing, paragliding, and river-rafting.

Sports Trivia

Who is Roger Federer?
A tennis pro. Roger Federer was the first Swiss man to win a Grand Slam title

What is *hornussen*?
A traditional Swiss game similar to baseball.

What is *steinstossen*?
Stone putting. The object of the game is to throw a stone weighing 184 pounds as far as possible.

How is Swiss wrestling, *schwingen*, played?
Each wrestler wears a pair of canvas-like shorts over his pants and tries to throw his opponent to the ground by grabbing hold of these shorts.

What is *jass*?
A popular game played with 36 cards.

Where are wrestling matches held?
In a ring filled with sawdust.

What happens at the end of a wrestling match?
The winner wipes the sawdust off the loser's shoulders to show good sportsmanship.

When did wrestling begin in Switzerland?

Schwingen dates back to at least 1200 AD when it was started by Swiss farmers and dairymen. After the chores of the day were done, they took turns wrestling to see who was the strongest.

What is *Unspunnen*?

A huge glacial boulder so heavy most people can't even lift it. The strongest men in Switzerland compete to see who can lift and throw it the farthest.

When did *Unspunnen* become a sport?

Unspunnen first became an organized sport at a festival to celebrate the departure of the French and Switzerland's freedom.

Game

I Spy Something. A group game.

Number of players. Two or more.

To play. Seat residents in a circle. The activity leader will then say, "I spy with my little eye something that is green." Then the residents take turns guessing what the leader has spotted in the room. The leader says "hot" or "cold" based on how close the guess is to the object.

Winner. The first person to guess the object wins and is the leader of the next round.

ICHI benefits. Mental benefits of language, speech, and articulation.

Music and Dance

Music

Think Switzerland and music, and you are likely to think of yodeling. However, yodeling is not a Swiss invention. Historians believe yodeling began during the early Stone Age in other parts of Europe including Poland. In Switzerland some believe yodeling comes from a form of long-distance communication and cow-calls.

Traditional Swiss musical instruments include the *alphorn*, *schwyzerorgeli*, *hackbrett*, and *trümpi*.

The *alphorn* is made from a conical bore with a wooden cup-shaped mouthpiece. Historians believe the horn originated in northern Asia and was brought to Europe by nomadic tribes. Originally used for call and sign, the *alphorn* was first used to play tunes at the end of the eighteenth century.

The *schwyzerörgeli* is a type of accordion, the *hackbrett* is a hammered dulcimer, and the *trümpi* is similar to a Jew's harp.

The recorded history of Swiss music began in 860 AD when Notker Balbulus, a monk at the monastery of St. Gallen, composed about 860 hymns called Sequences that became the most popular form of singing during the Middle Ages. This music was spread throughout the country by *minnesingers*, also called troubadors, during this same period.

Ludwig Senfl was a well-known composer of motets and masses in Latin during the late 1400s and early 1500s. Heinrich Loris was a music theorist who wrote about tuning modes.

In the twentieth century, the country produced well-known composers such as Arthur Honegger who wrote the opera *Antigone* in 1928 and Rolf Liebermann who wrote the opera *Penelope* in 1954, as well as works for orchestra and chamber music choirs.

The Swiss listen to many forms of music including classical, Swiss folk, rock and roll, and American country. The nation's national public radio, funded by listeners, is required to play a mix of music from jazz to pop hits. Surveys of this group show that about two-thirds of the Swiss prefer popular music and about 10 percent prefer alpine, folk, classical, and US-style country music.

Music Videos

Jodel Schweizer Militärmusik [Yodeling and music by Swiss Army
      Band]: Accessed January 20, 2015,
      https://www.youtube.com/watch?v=0dC1f6bdyr4
Schwyzerörgeli: Accessed January 20, 2015,
      https://www.youtube.com/watch?v=N7oo3JIu1BQ
Swiss Army Band, Alphorn and Nicolas Senn (hackbrett) Tattoo
      Aventicum Musical Parade: Accessed January 20, 2015,
      https://www.youtube.com/watch?v=OPIMTpJUJ68

Dance

Schuhplattler is a traditional Alpine dance that began as a courtship display by men to attract the attention of women. The dance was written about in 1050 by a monk of Tegernsee Abbey in the knightly poem Ruodlieb.

In the beginning, the dance style was free without rules. Usually performed in 3/4 time, a series of jumps and hip movements would be performed with the male dancers rhythmically striking their thighs, knees, and soles of their feet, clapping their hands, and stamping their feet.

The former partner dance is nowadays usually performed by men only, often in the context of traditional shows by Trachten societies which maintain Austro-Bavarian costumes and songs called Volksmusik. Today there are also female groups which perform the dance.

Dance Videos

Blumenauer Schuhplattler Oktoberfest 2013: Accessed March 15, 2015,
    https://www.youtube.com/watch?v=KNo_xzWGics
Gaflenzer Jubiläumsplattler 2011: Accessed March 15, 2015,
    https://www.youtube.com/watch?v=vrMnW4fo4dk
Schuplattler: Accessed March 15, 2015,
    https://www.youtube.com/watch?v=w5mRA3dE4hU

Music and Dance Trivia

What is the Swiss national anthem?
The *Swiss Psalm*.

Who is Mani Matter?
He is considered the father of all contemporary Swiss singer-songwriters. His adaptations of French-style chansons are very popular.

Who was Jean-Jacques Rousseau?
He was known as one of the most influential thinkers during the eighteenth-century European Enlightenment period. His book *A Discourse on the Arts and Sciences* discussed how science and arts had caused the corruption of virtue and morality. Rousseau was also a composer and music theorist.

Who was Notker Balbulus?
A monk from the famous monastery of St. Gallen who composed about 860 hymns which became the most popular form of singing in the Middle Ages.

Who were *minnesingers*?
Musicians performing during the medieval period.

Who was Ludwig Senfl?
A composer for the German emperor Maximilian and for Bavarian duke William IV. Senfl was the most prominent composer of polyphonic works in German language in the early sixteenth century.

Who was Heinrich Loris?
A poet and music theorist, remembered for his treatise *Dodecachordon*.

Who was Rolf Liebermann?
An opera manager in Paris and Hamburg who composed opera, orchestra, and chamber music.

How did the tradition of Swiss brass bands begin?
In the Swiss military.

True or false: American country music is popular in Switzerland.
True.

Food

The Swiss are light eaters. Breakfast typically includes bread, butter or margarine, marmalade or honey, cheese or cereal, plus cold or hot milk, cold or hot chocolate, tea, or coffee. Lunch is a sandwich or sometimes a full meal.

Dinner might be a full main course or just some bread, cheese, and dried meat, or any other light meal, washed down with beverages ranging from plain water to soft drinks or beers and wines as well as a variety of hot drinks including many flavors of tea and coffee.

Swiss food varies from region to region, influenced by the cuisines of Germany, Italy, and France. One favorite Swiss food is cheese fondue, eaten by placing a bread cube on a fork and then dipping it into melted cheese. *Raclette* is melted cheese served with *gschwellti* (jacket potatoes), cocktail gherkins, onions, and pickled fruit.

Älplermagronen is a mixture of potatoes, macaroni, cheese, cream, and onions with a stewed apple on the side. *Rosti* is a flat, hot cake made of grated potatoes, either cooked jacket or raw, and fried in hot butter or another fat.

Birchermüesli was created in 1900 by the Swiss doctor Maximilian Oskar Bircher-Brenner. It is a mixture of oat flakes, lemon juice, condensed milk, grated apples, and hazelnuts or almonds.

The food everyone thinks of when they think Switzerland is Swiss chocolate. This tasty dessert chocolate was brought to Europe in the sixteenth century and by the seventeenth century was being produced in Switzerland. In the second half of the nineteenth century Swiss chocolate had a reputation abroad, especially with the invention of milk chocolate by Daniel Peter as well as the development of conching, fondant chocolate, by Rodolphe Lindt.

Recipe

Swiss Chocolate Bars. A great dessert. Makes 36 servings.

Ingredients.
For the bars:
2 cups all-purpose flour
2 cups sugar
1 teaspoon baking soda
½ teaspoon salt
2 eggs
½ cup sour cream
1 cup water
½ cup butter
1½ ounces unsweetened chocolate
For the frosting:
4 cups confectioner's sugar
½ cup butter
⅓ cup milk
1½ ounces unsweetened chocolate
1 teaspoon vanilla extract
Pecan halves.

Preparation. In a large bowl, combine the flour, sugar, baking soda, and salt. In a small bowl, combine eggs and sour cream. In a small saucepan, cook and stir water, butter, and chocolate just until melted, then add to the dry ingredients. Stir in sour cream mixture until well blended.

Pour into a greased 15" x 10" baking pan. Bake at 375 degrees F. for 25 minutes or until a toothpick inserted near the center comes out clean. Cool on a wire rack for 30 minutes.

While the bars cool, make the frosting: Put the confectioner's sugar in a large bowl. In a small saucepan combine the butter, milk, and chocolate. Bring to a boil and stir constantly. Beat into confectioner's sugar until smooth. Stir in vanilla. Let stand for 5 minutes. Spread over warm bars. Top with pecan halves. Cool completely before cutting into bars.

Food Trivia

What is *vacherin*?
A soft cheese.

What is *magenbrot*?
Sweet pieces of bread often sold at street fairs.

What is *emmentaler*?
A cheese famous for its big holes.

When are *zimtsterne* (cinnamon cookies) served?
At Christmas.

What is *schokolade kuchen*?
A chocolate cake with chocolate and vanilla icing spread in the style of a spider web.

What is *nusstorte*?
Nut cake.

What is *tete de moine*?
A cheese which is shaped into rosettes.

How many kinds of cheese are produced in Switzerland?
About 450.

Where do farmers sell their cheese?
At the weekly farmers' markets.

Where can tourist see cheese produced?
During tours of local cheese cellars.

Customs

Weddings

A marriage ceremony in Switzerland begins at a government registry office in order to have the proper documents for a church or civil wedding.

The engagement ring is made of gold which symbolizes the financial sacrifice that the groom makes for his bride-to-be. These days the gold ring usually is set with a diamond.

Church weddings are usually an afternoon ceremony and include performances by the guests such as skits, playing music, and reading poetry. These events are coordinated by the maid-of-honor and best man.

As in the US, Swiss brides wear something old, something new, something blue, and something borrowed. Something old represents the continuity of tradition and can be a scarf or a piece of jewelry passed on from generation to generation. Something new stands for the future and hope and can be anything from the wedding band to clothing. Something borrowed indicates future happiness and is usually contributed by a happily married, close friend of the bride. Blue symbolizes purity and the couple tries to incorporate that color in their Swiss wedding outfit.

A Swiss bride wears a traditional crown or wreath of flowers on her head to represent maidenhood and youth. The wreath is removed and burned after the couple exchanges vows. A quick-burning crown means the bride will be lucky.

The old tradition of kidnapping the bride was needed in the past because the groom often had to fight the bride's angry relatives. This has become a fun game played by the bridal party and guests after the wedding.

Children

Babies do not sleep in bassinets but rather in *haengemattes*, hammocks that bounce, rock, and swing to soothe the baby. It is believed that this motion helps calm babies with colic.

Lichterschwemmen is the festival of floating lights that occurs on Ermensee Lake. In Untervaz boys and single men stand on a hill and throw red-hot wooden discs into the valley at the *Schiibaschlaha* ritual on the first Sunday in Lent. Each fiery disc is dedicated to a girl or an unmarried woman.

Another festival celebration for children is *Zwänzgerle*, an Easter egg game takes some skill and was designed to provide a bit of extra pocket money for the children. The children stand facing the adults, holding up hard-boiled decorated eggs. The adults throw small coins at the eggs with the goal of getting the coins to rest on the eggs. If the coin drops, the child keeps the egg and the coin, but if the Zwänzgerle coin stays on the egg, the person who threw it keeps the egg and the coin.

Holidays

January 1. New Year's Day
Variable date. Good Friday
Variable date. Easter
Variable date. Easter Monday
Variable date. Whit Monday
August 1. Swiss National Day
December 25. Christmas
December 26. St. Stephen's Day
December 31. New Year's Eve

Customs Trivia

Who leads the guests to the reception after the wedding ceremony?
A junior bridesmaid leads the procession to the reception and passes out colored handkerchiefs to the guests.

What do wedding guests give the bride?
Each guest gives a coin for the starting of the new home.

Why is the wedding ring worn on the ring finger of the left hand?
The Swiss believe this is the location of the love vein which will enhance the romance of the marriage.

True or false: Guests throw rice as the happy couple leave the church.
False: They throw small square sweetcakes called *zaltli*.

Why does the newly married couple plant a tree in their yard?
As a sign of fertility and future good luck.

What is a *baumstamm sagen*?
A log on a sawhorse placed in the couple's path as they exit the church. The couple must work together on a two-sided saw to cut the log in half as a sign they can work together during their marriage.

What do female wedding guests do the night before the wedding?
They meet to make bouquets for the wedding. They also make an extra bouquet as they may leave flowers on the doorstep of the man they love on their way home.

Why does the newly married couple walk on fir branches from the wedding site to their car?
To bring good luck to their first steps as husband and wife.

True or false: The tooth fairy is a mouse.
True. The Swiss follow the French custom of *la petite souris*, a mouse who leaves money for a lost tooth.

True or false: Babies in Switzerland are raised with strict routines for feedings and sleep.
True.

More Resources

DVDs

Crossing the Swiss Alps, DVD, Travelscope Instant video, 2007.
Culinary Travels Swiss Cheese, DVD, TravelVideoStore.com, 2006.
Rick Steves' Europe: Germany, Swiss Alps and Travel Skills, DVD,
    Avalon Travel Publishers, 2003.

Switzerland Country of Mountains, DVD, TravelVideoStore.com, 2013.
Travelview International Switzerland, DVD, TravelVideoStore.com, 2009.

Books

Fisher, T. 2012. *National Geographic Traveler: Switzerland* (National Geographic, 2012).

Foder's. *Foder's Switzerland Full-Color Travel Guide* (Fodor's, 2015).

Geography Department Lerner Publications. *Switzerland in Pictures* (Minneapolis: Lerner Publications, 1996).

Steves. R. *Rick Steves' Switzerland* (Avalon Travel Publishing; 2014).

Williams, N., Christiani, K., O'Brien, S., and Simoni, D. *Lonely Planet Switzerland Travel Guide* (Lonely Planet, 2012).

Websites

All About Switzerland: Accessed March 16, 2015, http://swiss-government-politics.all-about-switzerland.info/

Embassy of Switzerland in the United States of America: Accessed March 16, 2015, https://www.eda.admin.ch/eda/en/home/reps/nameri/vusa/wasemb.html

Flag of Switzerland 2015: Accessed January 18, 2015, http://www.worldflags101.com/s/switzerland-flag.aspx

Government of Switzerland. Useful links: Accessed March 16, 2015, http://www.oecd.org/general/governmentofswitzerlandusefullinks.htm

Swiss World. Tourism: Accessed March 16, 2015, http://www.swissworld.org/en/economy/key_sectors/tourism/

Photos

Nature and Landscape Photography: Accessed March 16, 2015, http://www.myswitzerland.com/en-us/nature-and-landscape-photography.html

Landscape in Switzerland: Accessed March 16, 2015,
   http://www.pbase.com/19sweetcorn92/landscape_in_switzerland&page=all

Swiss Alps Winter: Accessed March 16, 2015,
   http://funkystock.photoshelter.com/gallery/Swiss-Alps-Winter-Alpine-Pictures-Photos-Images-Fotos/G0000uvklR88aonQ/C0000DPgRJMSrQ3U

Switzerland Photo Gallery: Accessed March 16, 2015,
   http://travel.nationalgeographic.com/travel/countries/switzerland-photos-traveler/

Switzerland Pictures: Accessed March 16, 2015,
   http://www.tripadvisor.com/LocationPhotos-g188045-Switzerland.html

References

All About Switzerland: Accessed January 18, 2015, http://official-swiss-national-languages.all-about-switzerland.info/index.html

Brief History of Switzerland: Accessed January 18, 2015,
   http://www.nationsonline.org/oneworld/History/Switzerland-history.htm

Countries and Their Culture. Switzerland: Accessed March 15, 2015,
   http://www.everyculture.com/Sa-Th/Switzerland.html

Countries and Their Cultures. Swiss Americans: Accessed January 18, 2015,
   www.everyculture.com/multi/Sr-Z/Swiss-Americans.html#ixzz3PD6uFnm3

Culture, Heritage, Roots: Accessed January 18, 2015,
   http://theswisscenter.org/swissroots/

Discover Switzerland: Accessed January 18, 2015,
   http://www.swissworld.org/en/geography/rivers_and_lakes/water_sources/

Famous Birthdays: Accessed January 18, 2015,
   http://www.famousbirthdays.com/people/louis-chevrolet.html

Food in Switzerland: Accessed March 15, 2015,
   http://www.about.ch/culture/food/index.html#CH_EatDrink

Holidays in Switzerland: Accessed January 18, 2015,
   http://www.timeanddate.com/holidays/switzerland/

Hotels in Switzerland: Accessed March 15, 2015,
   http://www.travelmath.com/from/Seattle,+WA/to/Bern,+Switzerland

Interesting Facts About Switzerland: Accessed January 18, 2015,
   http://www.eupedia.com/switzerland/trivia.shtml

My Switzerland. Typical Food: Accessed March 15, 2015,
   http://www.myswitzerland.com/en-us/typical-food.html

Schuhplattler: Accessed March 15, 2015, http://en.wikipedia.org/wiki/Schuhplattler

Swiss Children's Games: Accessed January 19, 2015,
http://www.ehow.com/list_6788857_swiss-children_s-games.htmlhttp://www.ehow.com/list_6788857_swiss-children_s-games.html

Swiss Chocolate Bars Recipe: Accessed March 15, 2015,
http://www.tasteofhome.com/recipes/swiss-chocolate-bars

Swiss Traditions for Your Wedding: Accessed March 15, 2015,
http://www.greenbrideguide.com/blog/swiss-traditions-your-wedding

Switzerland: Accessed March 15, 2015, http://www.encyclopedia.com/topic/Swiss.aspx

Switzerland: Accessed March 15, 2015,
http://www.lonelyplanet.com/switzerland/sights/arts-culture-literary/stiftsbibliothek/item-a-1116274-id

Switzerland: Accessed January 18, 2015,
http://www.nationsencyclopedia.com/economies/Europe/Switzerland.html#ixzz3PCOLlX1Q

Switzerland. Fun Facts and Information: Accessed January 18, 2015,
http://www.funtrivia.com/en/Geography/Switzerland-382.html

Traditional Swiss Sports: Accessed March 15, 2015, http://easyscienceforkids.com/all-about-traditional-swiss-sports/

Travel Math Switzerland: Accessed March 15, 2015,
http://www.travelmath.com/from/Seattle,+WA/to/Bern,+Switzerland

Wedding Customs and Traditions in Switzerland: Accessed March 15, 2015,
http://www.premiumswitzerland.com/travel-news/weddings/wedding-traditions-in-switzerland.htm

WALES

Basics

Geography

Wales lies west of England and is separated from England by the Cambrian Mountains. It is bordered on the northwest, west, and south by the Irish Sea and on the northeast and east by England. It is about the size of New Jersey and is the home of Skokholm Island, the United Kingdom's first bird reserve, established in 1933. Other interesting landscapes of the country include Ogof Fynnon Ddu, the country's deepest cave at 1,010 feet, and the oldest tree, the Llangeryw Yew, estimated to be between 4,000 and 5,000 years old. Copper has been mined in the country's oldest mine at Parys Mountain for over 4,000 years.

Language

Everyone speaks English, however over 20 percent of the population, half a million people, also speak Welsh, which dates back to the sixth century and is one of Europe's oldest languages. Because the Welsh government officially recognizes the Welsh language, road signs and other public signage list information in both English and Welsh. Students are required to study Welsh through age 16 and there is a Welsh language radio and television station.

History

People have lived in Wales for over 230,000 years. Scientists believe the first settlers were Neanderthals. Homo sapiens arrived in about 31,000 BC. Continuous habitation by modern humans dates from around 9000 BC, the period after the end of the last Ice Age.

The first recorded history of the area was the arrival of the Romans in 1 AD. Trouble between Welsh tribes and Anglo-Saxons began in the eighth century. The Welsh won those early battles but lost to William the Conqueror and his Norman armies in 1093. By 1282 English control of Wales was complete and in 1284 the Statute of Rhuddlan formalized England's sovereignty over Wales. In 1301 King Edward I gave his son, the future Edward II, the title Prince of Wales, a gesture meant to indicate the unity and relationship between the two lands. With the exception of Edward II, all subsequent British monarchs have given this title to their eldest son.

In 1400 the Welsh prince Owen Glendower led a revolt against the English and won. However, in less than ten years, his rebellion was crushed and the country was again possessed by England. In 1485 Henry VII, who was a Welshman and the first in the Tudor line, became king of England. His reign, and those of subsequent Tudors, made English rule more palatable to the Welsh. His son King Henry VIII joined England and Wales under the Act of Union in 1536.

In 1999, with the strong support of Britain's Prime Minister Tony Blair, Wales established the Welsh national assembly, the first real Welsh self-government in more than 600 years.

Map and Flag

Flag of Wales: Accessed March 7, 2015,
    http://www.activityvillage.co.uk/wales-flag-colouring-page
Map of Wales: Accessed March 7, 2015,
    http://printablecolouringpages.co.uk/?s=map%20of%20wales

Travel

Distance

From New York, NY, to Cardiff is 3,344 miles. Flight time is 7 hours 11 minutes.

From Chicago, IL, to Cardiff is 3,840 miles. Flight time is 8 hours 11 minutes.

From Dallas, TX, to Cardiff is 4,639 miles. Flight time is 9 hours 47 minutes.

From Seattle, WA, to Cardiff is 4,717 miles. Flight time is 9 hours 56 minutes.

Hotels

Abbey Hotel. Located at 149-151 Cathedral Road, Cardiff, near Swalec Stadium, Cardiff University, and Millennium Stadium, it offers free WiFi as well as free breakfasts for guests.

Celtic Manor Resort. Located on Chepstow Road, Coldra Wood, Newport, in a regional park 1.6 miles from Isca Augusta and within six miles of University of Wales-Newport and Newport Cathedral, it features a full spa and a golf course.

Fox & Hounds. Located in Llancarfan Barry within six miles of Cottrell Park Golf Resort and Brynhill Golf Club, it is a historic inn featuring a full breakfast every morning.

Mercure Cardiff Holland House Hotel and Spa. Located at 24-26 Newport Road in Cardiff, a 15-minute walk from Capitol Shopping Centre, National Museum Wales, and Cardiff Castle.

Parc by Thistle. Located at Park Place, Cardiff, near the National Museum Wales and Millennium Stadium, it has 24-hour room service.

Landmarks

Cardiff Castle. In the heart of the capital city, it covers about 30 acres and is considered to be one of the greatest castles in the Western world, with its lavish murals, stained glass, and ornate gilding.

Castell Coch. A lavish estate in a natural setting, considered one of Wales' most romantic castles.

Castell Dinas Bran. Legends claim the Holy Grail is hidden under its 2,600-year-old ruins.

Colwyn Bay. In North Wales, it has one of the longest promenades anywhere in the UK as well as a thriving farmers market where the organic pork is reported to be especially good. Or you can catch your own dinner from the end of the pier.

Llandudno. This town is framed by a pair of limestone headlands, the Great Orme and the Little Orme, with two Blue Flag beaches in between and a perfectly preserved Victorian seafront.

Merthyr Mawr Warren. Location of some of the largest sand dunes in Europe, where the movie *Lawrence of Arabia* was filmed.

Snowdon Peak. In the heart of Snowdonia National Park, at 3,560 feet it is the highest peak in all of Wales and England.

Tenby. A coastal community with three beaches which stretch for three miles, made with arguably the most sandcastle-friendly sand in Britain.

Travel Trivia

Who was Bartholomew Roberts?
One of the most successful pirates, he created the pirate flag, the Jolly Roger, in 1721, raided over 750 ships, and held Sunday Services on his ship.

Who was Robert Recorde?
The court physician to Edward VI and Mary Tudor, he invented algebra's plus, minus, and equal signs.

Who was George Everest?
A geographer for whom Mt. Everest was named. He was knighted in 1861 and elected vice president of the Royal Geographical Society in 1862.

Who was Henry Morton Stanley?
An explorer famous for reportedly saying, "Dr. Livingstone, I presume," when he found explorer Dr. Robert Livingstone in Zanzibar.

What is the most famous Welsh town name?
Llanfairpwllgwyngyllgogerychwrndrobwllllantysiliogogogoch, meaning "St. Mary's Church in the hollow of the while hazel near to the rapid

whirlpool and the church of St. Tysilio of the red cave." The town's nickname is Llanfair PG.

Where is Llanfair PG?
On the Isle of Anglesy. It is the fifth largest settlement on the island.

Where was Prince Charles installed as Prince of Wales?
At Caernarfon Castle, on which construction was started in 1283 but never completed.

How old is the Prince of Wales ceremony?
It was first performed in 1301 with the naming of Edward II.

What is the symbol on the Welsh flag?
The Welsh Dragon has been depicted on the flag since 1959.

Why do the Welsh wear a leek or daffodil on March 1?
Both are Welsh emblems used to celebrate St. David's Day.

What Welsh railway is the model for the *Thomas the Tank Engine* series?
Talyllyn Railway.

What is the capitol of Wales?
Cardiff, also the biggest Welsh city, located in the biggest Welsh county.

Who is the patron saint of Wales?
St. David, who lived for 100 years and died on March 1, now a Welsh national holiday.

What is the smallest city in Wales?
St. Davids, on the western coast has a population of less than 1,500.

What is the longest river in Wales?
River Severn, 210 miles long and named for Sabrina, daughter of the mistress of King Locrine, who drowned after the queen threw her in the river.

What is the national flower?
The daffodil. Legend says that whoever sees the first daffodil of spring will be blessed with gold in the coming year.

What cat breed has a Welsh name?
Cymric, also called Longhaired Manx, even though the cat originated in North America.

What is the largest body of water?
Bala Lake.

What is the Welsh motto?
The Red Dragon Leads the Way.

Cardiff has the oldest shop of its kind — what is it?
Spillers, a record store located on the Hayes, it was established in 1894 and began by selling sheet music.

America's Roots

Who was Daniel Boone?
An American pioneer born in Stonersville, Pennsylvania. In 1734 he led the exploration of Kentucky. He served three terms in the Virginia legislature and fought in the last battle of the Revolutionary War. His father came from Wales.

Who was Oliver Evans?
A visionary inventor, he created the grain elevator and various devices to automate the milling of flour, and went on to design the first fully automated industrial process, America's first high-pressure steam engine, and the very first amphibious vehicle and American automobile. In 1790 he received the third patent granted in the US. He was born in Delaware of Welsh descent.

Who was George Jones?
The co-founder of the New York Times newspaper along with Henry Jarvis Raymond on September 18, 1851. He insisted on a buffer between advertising and editorials and set a high standard for journalists' integrity. He was of Welsh descent.

Who was Meriwether Lewis?
The leader of the Lewis and Clark Expedition which explored the Louisiana Purchase starting in 1803 and reached the Pacific Coast in 1805. He became governor of the Louisiana Territory in 1808. His father is of Welsh ancestry.

Who was Daniel Morgan?
A brigadier general in the Continental Army during the American Revolution, he served in the US House of Representatives for Virginia. Born in New Jersey, his grandparents were from Wales.

Who was William Penn?
The founder of Pennsylvania. Born in England, he had Welsh ancestors and helped the Welsh members of the Society of Friends escape persecution and find religious freedom.

Who was Thomas Jefferson?
The third US President and a writer of the Declaration of Independence. He traced Welsh ancestry to his mother's family.

Who was Robert Morris?
The foremost financier of the American Revolution and a signer of the Declaration of Independence. He had Welsh ancestors.

Who was Gouverneur Morris
He wrote the final draft of the US Constitution. He was born in New York and had Welsh ancestors.

Who was John Marshall?
The fourth US Chief Justice and the father of American constitutional law. He was born in Virginia and had Welsh ancestors.

Who was John L. Lewis?
An American leader of organized labor who served as president of the United Mine Workers of America (UMW) from 1920 to 1960. He was born in a Welsh settlement in Iowa.

Who were Joseph and David Richards?
The Richards brothers co-founded the Knoxville Iron Works. They convinced 104 Welsh immigrants living in Pennsylvania to relocate to work in their business.

Who was Frank Lloyd Wright?
A world-famous architect, interior designer, writer, and educator, who designed more than 1,000 structures. His designs were called organic architecture because they were constructed in harmony with the environment. He was born in Wisconsin and his mother was from Wales.

Who was Lorin Morgan-Richards?
Founder of the Welsh League of Southern California in 2014. He was born in Wales and moved to America in the 1900s.

What TV show features a fictional American town with a Welsh name?
One Life to Live was set in Llanview, Pennsylvania. *Llan* is an old Welsh word for *church*.

Sports and Games

Sports

The Welsh love sports. With a capacity of 74,500, the Millennium Stadium in Cardiff is the largest stadium in Europe to feature a fully retractable roof. In 2014 the city of Cardiff was chosen as the European Capital of Sport.

The most popular sport is rugby, followed by boxing, cricket, and football. Golf is also very popular. The world's third largest sporting event, the Ryder Cup, a golf tournament, was held at the Celtic Manor Resort in Newport, Wales, in 2010. The Celtic Manor is one of Europe's leading golf resorts and a perennial stop on golf's European Tour. There are over 200 golf courses in the country. In addition, Wales has hosted international cricket games including the 2009 Ashes Test Opener.

Wales has produced internationally known sports stars including footballer Gareth Bale and taekwondo Olympic gold medalist Jade Jones. Thirty Welsh Olympic competitors and 8 Welsh Paralympic competitors took part in the 2012 Olympics. Team Wales has also been very successful at competing in the Commonwealth Games, winning a record-breaking 36 medals at the Glasgow 2014 Commonwealth Games, including 5 gold medals. Rhythmic gymnast Frankie Jones won six medals at the games plus the David Dixon Award which recognizes an outstanding athlete at the Commonwealth Games.

Sports Trivia

What is rugby?
A full-contact sport resembling American football. Matches are 80 minutes long with two 40-minute halves. The field is similar in size to a football or soccer field.

How big is a rugby ball?

Bigger and more oblong than an American football, it is 11 to 13 inches long, weighing 13.5 to 15.5 ounces.

How did the game of rugby begin?

According to legend, rugby was created in 1823 at Rugby School in Warwickshire. Apparently during a student football (soccer) game, William Webb Ellis picked up the ball and started running with it.

Who invented lawn tennis?

Major Walter Clopton Wingfield of Llanelldan, Denbighshire, in 1873.

Why the unusual shape of rugby balls?

Rugby balls are oval because they used to be made of pig bladders which are oval-shaped when inflated.

What is a *try* in rugby?

A *try* is scored by grounding the ball on or behind the opposition's goal line. The term comes from *try at goal*, originally meaning that grounding the ball gave the opportunity to try to score with a kick at goal.

What is a *sin bin*?

If a rugby player misbehaves resulting in receiving a yellow card, he or she is sent to the *sin bin*, a place on the sideline to think about what they have done for 10 minutes!

Rugby is the national sport of what three countries?

Wales, Madagascar, and New Zealand.

True or false: Basketball is said to have been started by a rugby coach in 1891.

True. He wanted an indoor sport to keep his players fit during the winter.

Where is the best place for bog snorkeling?

Llanwrtyd Wells.

Game

Conkers. Based on a fifteenth-century game using hazelnuts, Conkers has been played since 1848. The origin of the name is unknown, but some believe is comes from the French word *cogner*, meaning *to hit*.

Number of players. An even number of players. each with a conker. This could be played in residents' rooms as a one-on-one ice breaker for visitors.

Materials. The traditional conker is a nut from the horse chestnut tree, but this can be adapted by using a Ping-pong ball for each player, 6" string for each ball, and a drill. Drill a hole through the ball, thread the string through the hole and tie to secure.

To play. Two players each have a conker. During the game, one player holds out his conker so that it dangles in the air on the string. The goal of the game is for the other player to hit the first player's conker with his own.

Winner. Players take turns until one is successful or they may play until one player has 20 hits.

ICHI benefits. Cognitive language, speech and math skills, physical voluntary control of movements, hand and eye coordination, mobility of joints, and muscle tone.

Music and Dance

Music

Wales has been called "The Land of Song." Its history of vocal music began in the eighteenth century with the rise of the Methodist movement in which singing hymns was an important part of the experience. Congregational singing gained momentum with the rise of the temperance movement in the early part of the nineteenth century when annual festivals for singing were established.

Hymns are popular at rugby matches. Often called *Bread of Heaven*, *Guide Me O Thou Great Redeemer* is known as the Welsh rugby hymn.

A *Gymanfa Ganu* is a singing festival that involves a congregation singing sacred hymns in four-part harmony in Welsh, conducted by a choral director or choir master. The annual Cymanfa Ganu is a key event at the National Eisteddfod of Wales.

Many male choirs had their roots in the competitive choral singing and heavy industry of the nineteenth century. Often a group of miners working together would form a choir to enter a competition or *eisteddfod* and then disband shortly after. Other choirs thrived and survived, such as the Treorchy and Morriston Orpheus choirs, now famous throughout the world.

Although male choirs seem to be particularly associated with Wales, female and mixed choirs are equally popular, and these days singing in a choir is increasingly recognized for the benefits of health and wellbeing.

Cerdd dant or *penillion* singing is a traditional style of singing in which poetry is sung to one tune against the accompaniment on a harp to a different tune. Until the middle of the twentieth century, *cerdd dant* was sung by individuals and was very much an improvised performance, mostly sung by men. Today you may hear duets, trios, parties, or choirs singing *cerdd dant* and the majority of singers are female.

Another Welsh singing tradition is *plygain*, men singing Welsh carols in rural churches from 3 am to 6 am on Christmas Day. This tradition dates back to the eighteenth century, has largely died out, but continues in Montgomeryshire.

Music Videos

Four Welsh Hymns. Cowbridge Male Voice Choir: Accessed March 9, 2015, https://www.youtube.com/watch?v=JyuVoea7mPo
Here is Love Vast as the Ocean: Accessed March 9, 2015, https://www.youtube.com/watch?v=APrUPPC8bFY
Welsh Hymn Singing: Accessed March 9, 2015, https://www.youtube.com/watch?v=Y6UZF8_BQLg&list=PLE8C75 86100590F90

Dance

Dance in Wales began thousands of years ago as folk dances. Clog dancing was originally performed by farmers and slate quarry workers in a competition where dancers would show off their stamina and athleticism. The difference between Welsh clogging and other step dance traditions is that the performance will not only include complicated stepping, but also tricks such as toby stepping which requires the dancer to make high leaps

The folk dancing tradition almost died out during the eighteenth and nineteenth centuries when the Methodist movement proclaimed folk arts and customs to be sinful. Thomas Charles and other preachers tried to stamp out dancing and folk singing, replacing them with hymn singing and chapel music.

Welsh dance culture was saved by William Jones, Edward Jones, and others who recorded dances on paper, including Welsh dances such as *meillionen* and *abergenni* which were created in the mid-seventeenth century.

Many Welsh dances became part of British/English collections, tending to keep their original Welsh names translated into English. For example, the dance *Hoffedd ap Hywel* became Powell's Fancy. The rich, lively Welsh folk culture gradually vanished, with only the odd clogger continuing to step and pass the tradition on to the next generation and with triple harpers still playing traditional tunes, many of which were dance tunes, in the mansions.

In the 1940s Lois Blake and Gwyn Williams began reviving the Welsh dancing tradition and in 1949 the Welsh Folk Dance Society was formed with the aim of promoting and resurrecting the old dances. There are now over 20 adult teams and many hundreds of school teams and Urdd clubs across Wales. The Urdd National Eisteddfod promotes Welsh dancing and attracts thousands of young people participating in dancing competitions every year.

Dance Videos

The Culture of Wales: Accessed April 2, 2015,
    https://www.youtube.com/watch?v=odoBFopH9NY
Welsh Folk Dancing at The National Eisteddfod, Swansea 2006:
    Accessed April 2, 2015,
    https://www.youtube.com/watch?v=pIOS19WzEZM
Welsh Traditional Dance: Accessed April 2, 2015,
    https://www.youtube.com/watch?v=LncCCxaATso

Music and Dance Trivia

Who is William Williams?
He wrote the hymn *Guide me, O Thou great Redeemer* which has been translated into 75 languages.

Who is Joseph Parry?
He composed the hymns *Myfanwy* and *Aberystwyth*, which are still sung today.

What is the *Mari Lwyd*?
Meaning *the Grey Mare*, it is a form of Welsh wassailing tradition in which a group of men carry a cloaked hobbyhorse house-to-house while singing and challenging the families inside to a battle of rhyming insults in Welsh. At the end of the battle of wits, known as *pwnco*, the group would be invited into the house for refreshments.

What is a popular Welsh bedtime song?
All Through the Night, written by Sir Harold Boulton in 1884.

What are the lyrics to *All Through the Night*?
Sleep, my child, and peace attend thee
All through the night.
Guardian angels God will send thee
All through the night.

Soft the drowsy hours are creeping,
Hill and vale in slumber sleeping,
I my loving vigil keeping
All through the night.

Who is Tom Jones?
A popular singer of the 1965 number-one hits *It's Not Unusual* and *What's New Pussycat*. His TV show *This is Tom Jones* aired in the US and UK from 1969 to 1971.

Who was Richard Burton
An actor and movie star from Wales.

Who is Anthony Hopkins?
An actor and movie star from Wales.

Who was Ivor Barry?
A Welsh film and television actor who served in the British Royal Artillery.

Who was Rosemarie Frankland?
A beauty pageant contestant who won the 1961 Miss United Kingdom and Miss World titles before becoming an actress.

Food

Native Welsh foods include seaweed, lamb, and cheeses. Popular dishes include Welsh cakes, a type of scone cooked on a stove-top griddle, and *bara brith*, or speckled bread, a wonderful sticky fruitcake smothered in butter and often served with afternoon tea.

Laverbread, not actually bread at all as it is made of seaweed, is often fried into crisp patties with eggs, bacon, and fresh cockles for a traditional Welsh breakfast.

Mineral water from Wales is sold around the world. Llanllyr Water is drawn from certified organic land in west Wales, a farm which has been in the same family for 800 years. Radnor Hills Water comes from the mountains of mid-Wales and is sold as far away as Malaysia and Australia and has won the coveted Queens Award for International Trade.

The first canned beer was invented in 1933 at the Felinfoel Brewery, Llanelli and was first offered for sale in 1935. There are over 250 Brains pubs across South Wales, the West Country, and central Cardiff.

The world's smallest commercial brewery is Bragdy Gwynant, located just outside Aberystwyth. It is less than five square feet in size and has just one customer, the next-door pub *The Tynllidiart Arms* where customers can enjoy good food made with local ingredients alongside their local pint.

Wales' 60 cider producers make about 1.1 million liters of cider per year, including Gwynty Ddraig which also produces *perry* and exports to Australia, Finland, Norway, and Germany.

Recipe

Bara Brith is a tea bread served topped with butter. Serves 12.
Ingredients.
Two tea bags
11 ounces boiling water
8 ounces mixed dried fruit
6 ounces self-rising white flour
6 ounces wholewheat flour
1 teaspoon baking powder
1 teaspoon ground allspice
2 ounces light dark brown sugar

1 beaten egg

Preparation. Place the tea bags in a heatproof measuring bowl and pour in boiling water. Stir and let sit for four minutes. Remove the tea bags and add dried fruit to the bowl. Squeeze the tea bags over the fruit. Cover and let the mix sit for five hours.

Preheat oven to 325 degrees F. Grease a two-pound loaf pan. In a large bowl, sift together the flours, baking powder, sugar, and spice. Pour in the soaked fruit and tea and stir. Add the beaten egg and mix together. Pour the batter into loaf pan and bake for 1½ hours. Remove from the pan and cool for 5-20 minutes prior to serving.

Food Trivia

What is Seaweed Gin?
An alcoholic beverage made from seaweed by the Dà Mhìle Distillery in Ceredigion, West Wales.

What is Orange 33?
An orange citrus alcoholic beverage.

Who produces sparkling wine in Wales?
Ancre Hill Estates

Where is the oldest vineyard in Wales?
Llanerch Vineyard in the Glamorgan countryside.

What is the Welsh word for pancakes?
Crempogen, which are served for both breakfast and dessert.

Name two food exports from Wales.
Welsh whisky and sea salt.

What is Glamorgan sausage?
A vegetarian dish using Caerphilly cheese and leeks.

What is *caw*?
A thick broth.

What is Welsh *rarebit*?
Traditionally, beef or roasted cod served on toast, sometimes with a poached egg on top.

What is the traditional Welsh Sunday meal?
Roast lamb.

Customs

Weddings

The wedding day begins with capturing the bride. The groom and his friends go to the bride's house where they find the door locked. The groom must convince the bride's relatives to let him into the house where the bride is hiding. When the bride is found, the wedding party goes to the church. Then the father and brothers of the bride capture her and ride off. The groom catches up and wins his bride, and then they all return to the church for the wedding.

The *gwahoddwr*, or bidder, formally invites guests to the wedding and to the parents' home where the guests donate money to the couple.

Lavender is a lucky color for a wedding gown and black gowns are signs of bad luck. Tossing red clover blooms in the path of the bride will make her a woman of good taste.

Children

Many ancient Welsh beliefs center on children. A child born at sunrise will be clever, and one born in the afternoon or at sunset will be lazy. A child weaned at the time that birds migrate will be restless and changeable throughout life. If a babe is suckled again after being weaned it will become a profane adult.

Babies washed in rainwater talk earlier than they would otherwise. For the first three months of life, if the water in which a baby is washed is not thrown under a green tree, the babe will not thrive.

Holidays

January 1. New Year's Day
February 14. St. Valentine's Day
March 1. St. David's Day
Third Sunday in May, Mothering Sunday

Variable date. Good Friday
Variable date. Easter Monday
Third Sunday in June. Father's Day
Last Monday in August. Summer Bank holiday
Last Monday in September. Autumn Holiday
December 25. Christmas
December 26. Boxing Day
December 31. New Year's Eve

Customs Trivia

Where was the mythical King Arthur said to live?
Two sites are claimed to be the home of fortress Camelot, Geoffrey of
Monmouth and Chretien de Troyes, both in Caerleon.

What does the appearance of a load of hay in front of you mean?
You will have good luck.

How can you create good luck for yourself?
On Easter morning drawing water from a spring into a jug and then
throwing the water on the surrounding plants and shrubs ensures that you
will have good luck during the year.

What wild animal is unlucky only if seen in a group?
To see several foxes together is unlucky. If you see a single fox, you will
have good luck.

How can you make your wishes come true?
Make a cap out of hazel leaves and twigs and then wear it.

How can you have a successful voyage?
Throw a penny over the ship's bow when leaving dock.

How can you share good luck?
If anything from one ship is lent to another, luck goes with it.

How can you keep your household healthy?
A roof covered with houseleeks, a succulent perennial that forms mats of
rosettes of tufted leaves, ensures prosperity and protects the household
from disease.

How can you keep your family fed?
If you move from one home to another at the time of the new moon, you will have plenty of bread to spare.

How can you keep your money safe?
Money washed in clear rainwater cannot be stolen.

More Resources

DVDs

Rick Steve's England and Wales, DVD, Perseus, 2009.

Books

Campbell, K. *United Kingdom in Pictures* (Lerner Publications, 2004).
Williams. D. *Landscape Wales* (Graffeg, Peter Gill & Associates, 2010).

Websites

Visit Wales: Accessed December 29, 2015, www.visitwales.com.uk/
Welcome to gov.uk: Accessed December 29, 2015. www.direct.gov.uk/

Photos

Photos of Wales: Accessed December 29, 2015,
    http://www.urban75.org/photos/wales Wales
Photos: Accessed December 29, 2015,
    http://travel.nationalgeographic.com/travel/countries/wales-united-kingdom-photos/#/wales-whitesand-beach_3265_600x450.jpg
Wales Pictures: Accessed December 29, 2015,
    http://www.tripadvisor.com/LocationPhotos-g186425-Wales.html
Wales Pictures & Images: Accessed December 29, 2015,
    http://photobucket.com/images/wales

References

Ar Hyd y Nos [All Through the Night]: Accessed December 29, 2015,
    https://en.wikipedia.org/wiki/Ar_Hyd_y_Nos
Daniel Boone: Accessed December 29, 2015,
    https://en.wikipedia.org/wiki/Daniel_Boone
Geography and Map of the United Kingdom: Accessed December 29, 2015,
    http://geography.about.com/library/cia/blcuk.htm
Henry Morgan Stanley: Accessed December 29, 2015,
    https://en.wikipedia.org/wiki/Henry_Morton_Stanley
Interesting Animals Found in Wales: Accessed December 29, 2015, http://gypsy-
    willow.hubpages.com/hub/Interesting-Animals-Found-in-Wales_1
Interesting Facts About Wales: Accessed December 29, 2015,
    http://www.eupedia.com/wales/trivia.shtml
Meriwether Lewis: Accessed December 29, 2015,
    https://en.wikipedia.org/wiki/Meriwether_Lewis
Oliver Evans Biography (1755-1819): Accessed December 29, 2015,
    www.madehow.com/inventorbios/26/Oliver-Evans.html
Robert Recorde: Accessed December 29, 2015,
    https://en.wikipedia.org/wiki/Robert_Recorde
Tom Jones: Accessed December 29, 2015,
    www.infoplease.com/biography/var/tomjones.html
The New York Times Company: Accessed December 29, 2015,
    https://en.wikipedia.org/wiki/The_New_York_Times_Company
Traditional Welsh Food: Accessed December 29, 2015,
    http://www.squidoo.com/traditional-welsh-food
Welsh Americans: Accessed December 29, 2015,
    http://en.m.wikipedia.org/wiki/List_of_Welsh_Americans#section_1

Also by Gloria Hoffner

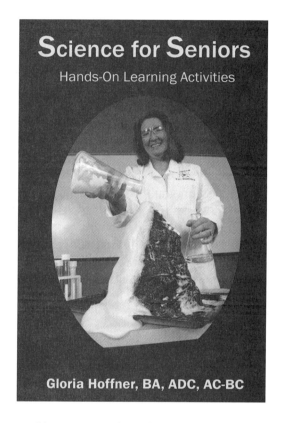

Science for Seniors
Hands-On Learning Activities

Gloria Hoffner, BA, ADC, AC-BC

… includes everything you need to know to develop a diverse science program… a helpful resource for the activity professional and recreational therapist.

Debbie Hommel, ACC/MC/EDU, CTRS

Gloria's vast knowledge of the field and her hands-on experience shows on every page… Everyone benefits from her enthusiasm and talent.

Nancy Newman, Activity Director, Sterling Healthcare and Rehab Center

Trade Paper, 288 pages, 6" by 9", ISBN 9781882883776, Price $28.00
Available at idyllarbor.com and you favorite online bookstores.

ABOUT THE AUTHOR

Gloria Hoffner is an award-winning activity professional and a career journalist. In 2010, *Science for Seniors* was awarded first place in Best Practice division of the National Certification Council of Activity Professionals. The award recognized *Science for Seniors* as the most outstanding new activity program design among retirement, assisted living, personal care, long-term care, and adult day center facilities. Gloria is a contributing editor and monthly columnist for *Creative Forecasting Magazine* and a columnist on activity program ideas for about.com. She is also a frequent speaker at international, national, and statewide conventions for professionals in the healthcare, activity, and certified therapeutic recreation fields. Gloria lives in Upper Providence, Pennsylvania, with her husband Jim.